The Pink Duck

"Surviving the Cancer Journey"

By

Karen Miller Weber

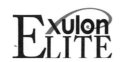

Copyright © 2015 by Karen Miller Weber

The Pink Duck
Surviving the Cancer Journey
by Karen Miller Weber

Printed in the United States of America.

ISBN 9781498428453

All rights reserved solely by the author. The author guarantees all contents are original and do not infringe upon the legal rights of any other person or work. No part of this book may be reproduced in any form without the permission of the author. The views expressed in this book are not necessarily those of the publisher.

Scripture quotations taken from the New International Version (NIV). Copyright © 1973, 1978, 1984, 2011 by Biblica, Inc.™. Used by permission. All rights reserved.

Scripture quotations taken from the King James Version (KJV) – *public domain*

www.xulonpress.com

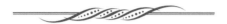

Dedicated to my sister Lynn who fought the brave fight to the end.
June 19, 1954 – August 18, 2002

Pray Today
If you do nothing else today,
At least take time to read and pray.
One day goes by so quick and fast:
What if today should be your last?
Down by your bedside, in earnest prayer
It needn't keep you there all day.
But get in touch with God on high,
Let Him know you're there and why.
You won't regret you took the time
When up the mountain side you climb.
You'll be glad you asked for strength
When the battle rages on at length.
And when the day comes to an end,
By your bedside kneel again.
Thank God for strength He gave that day,
That kept you going on the way.
Express your joy, your thanks, your love,
And God will bless you from above…
Then as you're drifting off to sleep
God will your trusting spirit keep!
By Lynn Segar

Preface

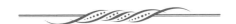

I love people! I love to watch people! I love to know their stories. I want to know why they are like they are and what causes the wrinkles and laugh lines around their eyes! I want to know why their eyes are sad! I want to sit by them and find out what makes them tick. Maybe that is what inspired me to spill and share so much of my guts in this book, I really don't know.

Early on in my journey our son Wesley started a Facebook page that would allow me to share some of my experiences with friends and family. Because our three sons are in different states and so much of our family lives at a distance, he felt like Facebook would be a good way to keep everyone informed of my cancer journey. As I shared, more and more of you encouraged me to write my story to help encourage and inspire others.

It is my prayer, if you are facing cancer or another disease that my story will help and inspire you. If a friend or a loved one has cancer or is fighting for their life in another way, I hope my story will give you a little insight of what some of us go through. Maybe it will show you how to inspire and encourage your loved one to keep fighting. In any case, I hope you get a few belly laughs as you journey along with me! Thank you for choosing to read my story! Please get yourself a PINK DUCK!!!

Acknowledgement

I wish to thank each and every one of you who encouraged me on my journey!

For each of you who prayed for me, whether it was one prayer or you were constantly praying for me. I especially want to thank those who are still praying for me!

I want to thank those who brought us meals and helped keep our home clean.

For those who kept us in fire wood all winter long! For our neighbors who never tired of helping. For those who helped when our water froze this winter! For our church family who supported us in blessings. For our community who pulled together and helped us.

My fear is if I began naming names, I will forget someone! I also want to thank each one who sent me special messages, cards, text and phone calls and those who encouraged me over and over to write this book. I think you had more faith than I did! A special thank you to each of you who brought potato soup! For my group of "besties" who propped me up and helped mop me up when the tears flowed!

Not one thing that you did for us went unnoticed or unappreciated!

A big shout out to my Doctors and nurses who stood by me and kept me in an upright position more than once. DR Voight, (surgeon) DR Nevils, (oncologist) DR Graham (radiation) and DR Cathy Bond who directed me on to the roller coaster ride. (Do not pass go…do not collect $200) My special nurses, who were there with encouragement more times than I can count. Carol Walters, Julie Terry, Stephanie Pritchett, Hillary Bleckman and Diana Panteleo helped me saddle up the bull and ride. A special thanks to Kent and Michelle who kept the Dragon at bay with gospel music and encouraging me to lie still!

A special thanks to my parents! Roy and Alice Miller

As parents do, you were there for me! Thank you for the nights I spent at your house! For staying up all night when I was high on chemo and for the biscuits and gravy!

Thank you to my sweet baby sister Jill Neugebauer (see I spelled it right Jill)

This gal never left my side! Thank you for every home made card made just for the occasion! For chocolate candy and warm socks! Thank you for my beautiful memory books! I'll cherish them forever!

Thank you to my sister-in-law Theresa Robinett who came and spent seven weeks with me. She is a cancer survivor and knew just when to laugh and when to cry with me!

Thank you to my three sons! Timothy, Wesley and James.

You know, I could not have survived this journey without your love and encouragement!

Thank you to Alexis and Melody Weber (aka Thing One and Thing Two)

You lit up my days in ways only precious granddaughters can do. You are my sunshine and I love you both to the moon and back along with Gabriella, Joshua, Abigail and Bethany! (My out of state sweet grandchildren)

Thank you to my Man! My Joe! You carried me way beyond the "for better or worse, through sickness and health!" You gave me courage when I had none. You made me feel beautiful bald and helped me keep my chin up! Never once did you complain! I know you'll never again ask me what the pink ducks are doing in the tub!! I love you forever and I'm proud to be your girl!!

Contents

Chapter 1	September: The Bubble Bath 13
Chapter 2	October: Hopping on the Roller Coaster 18
Chapter 3	November: Hair Today, Gone Tomorrow 26
Chapter 4	December: Bull Riding Gone Wild. 43
Chapter 5	January: Chop! Chop! The Chopping Block! 58
Chapter 6	February: Back On the Bull (It's anything but normal) 85
Chapter 7	March: Bone-tired, Bald and Water Logged! 102
Chapter 8	April: Happy Birthday to Me! 39 Plus Tax and Shipping 122
Chapter 9	May: Just Cleaning Up My Plate! 133
Chapter 10	June: Normal Isn't Normal Any More 150
Chapter 11	July: Facing the Monster 156
Chapter 12	August: Slaying the Dragon 166
Chapter 13	September: Coming Full Circle Makes Me Dizzy! 174
Chapter 14	October: Time to Kick Up My Heels & Pay It Forward. 184
Chapter 15	November: Thanksgiving. 189
Chapter 16	December: Chicken Soup & Pink Ducks . . .197

Chapter 1

The Bubble Bath

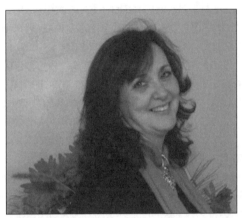

**February 2013 I really did have hair!!!
Before the journey started!!! No clue at this time!!**

Early September 2013

I slid down further into the warm water and stirred up some more bubbles with my foot. I watched the little pink duck bobble on the frothy bubbles and wondered how many little pink ducks I had passed out to people over the years. Hundreds! I would dare to say! I bought them by the bags full and passed them out to people to put them in their shower as a reminder to do their monthly exam. It worked for me and I hoped it worked for others.

I knew I had a lump of sorts, but I was convinced I was drinking too much caffeine and eating too much chocolate. I had cut back on both and was waiting to see what happened.

The little pink duck bobbled again and went under this time. I rescued him and set him upright and then grabbed the bar of soap.

The easiest way to do a self- exam is soaping up real good as you will be able to feel lumps, if any, easier. I'd had my share of lumps over the years but this one was aggravating me for some reason. I'd watched it a bit. It seemed to move easily but it wasn't going down and quite frankly I was getting tired of skipping the caffeine and chocolate!

I hopped out of the tub and stood with bubbles dripping, before the mirror. It was at that time I knew I was in for a bit of trouble. How much trouble I didn't know but I knew enough about the signs of breast cancer to know that if your breast puckers or turns in, you'd better head to the doctor.

Other than an occasional mammogram over the years, I probably hadn't been in a doctor's office three times in ten years! I wasn't a frequent visitor and wasn't inclined to go! I took my vitamins and cured headaches with chocolate and a Cola. If I ever got a cold, I used my mom's no fail, vinegar, garlic and honey recipe. Neither remedy had failed me yet.

It took me a week or so to get my courage up to call the doctor. When I called and told them I had a lump they got me right in. In fact, faster than my courage would have allowed. DR Cathy Bond gave me a good check over and asked me when I could schedule a mammogram.

Now, I'm a "Martha" personality. My date book is always full and I like it that way. I grabbed my book and looked at my next convenient date and told her I could come back in a month. She considered my answer and said: "That won't work. Go ahead and get dressed and I'll be back in a minute." I took my flowing pink cape off, folded it and put my street clothes back on. It didn't take long and Dr. Bond came in telling me I had a mammogram scheduled for one hour later! Now that made me nervous!

I didn't like the pictures on the mammogram screen even though I didn't really know what to look for. When they announced to me that I was being held for a sonogram and possibly a biopsy; I called my husband (Joe) who was in a meeting about a hundred miles away and told him my concerns. He left his meeting and headed my way and got there just in time for me to go in for the biopsy. At this time they went ahead and put in titanium markers.

Even though they had him sit across the room, I was comforted by the fact that he would come running when I was so worried. A comfort that he has continued to give me through this incredible journey I have embarked upon.

Here I sat in another "boost your confidence gown"! In one day... I had gone in to see my doctor to set up a mammogram, gone for a mammogram, had a sonogram, a biopsy and had titanium markers put in me (just in case I had surgery) Now I was being introduced to Breast Cancer Nurse Navigator Carol Walters... just in case! My world was beginning to spin! Afterwards, we went home to wait for results! But we didn't wait long!

September 23, 2013

A few days later, I was called to return to the doctor's office. Joe went with me to hold my hand. In my heart, I already knew what she was going to say before she walked through the door and looked me in the eyes. I expected the words, but I didn't have a clue about the journey!! Her eyes had tears in them as she explained to me that my test results weren't good and that I did indeed have cancer. And so.... I hopped on the cancer rollercoaster, just like that.

I hope to share my journey with you in a way that will both inspire and educate. Many people are unaware of the struggles that take place during a cancer journey. I know for myself, I had no idea what one would really face. I don't grasp medical terms easily. My theory in life has always been the K.I.S.S system. (Keep it simple sweetie) Grab a cup of coffee, tea or hot chocolate, pull up a chair and prop your feet. Let me see your precious face and tell you my story! Here it is!

We left the clinic and I called my little sister (Jill) and asked her to meet us at the park. Since we had already lost our big sister (Lynn) to ovarian cancer 11 years earlier; I knew my announcement of breast cancer was going to hit the family pretty hard. I let her know that I was ok with my diagnosis and we headed over to our parents' house to make our announcement.

I had decided that no matter what the outcome, we were going to celebrate and have a party! Family members gathered together to hear my diagnosis and we ordered pizza in. We didn't celebrate that I had good news. Instead, we celebrated that they had found the cancer and it was going to be taken care of. It was like an out of body experience! I went through the motions but my brain certainly wasn't functioning!

We called our three sons who were living in other states. They put together a Face book page for me to share my progress to keep my family and friends updated. In just five days, I had started down a path, not knowing where I was headed. I didn't know what to think, I didn't know what to feel! I was numb! Come! Go with me! I don't want to go alone!!

September 25, 2013

Anger hit me last night as I brushed my teeth and watched myself in the mirror...I gritted my teeth and said... "THIS is NOT what I had planned!" Tears slid down my cheeks! Immediately that verse from Jeremiah 29:11 came to me, "For I know the plans I have for you," declares the LORD, "plans to prosper you and not to harm you, plans to give you hope and a future."

This morning as I left to pick up Thing One and Thing Two... (My two little granddaughters) there was a huge bright double rainbow over my path!! So many are messaging me about what is going on and it's not that I've been trying to hide it. I just needed to let some family members know before putting it all out there.

I found out yesterday that I DO have breast cancer. Please keep praying for me and I'll keep appreciating your prayers and support. I have done things on my own and I have done things with the support of friends and family and it's so much easier to have the support of friends and family! I'm choosing YOU!

I've already had my visit with the Nurse Navigator (Carol Walters) who will guide me in this. I see the surgeon on Monday to schedule my surgery. I asked Nurse Carol if I could swim after this was over and she said yes!!! I told her I was excited about that because I can't swim now!!!

Thing Two told on me tonight!!! She complained to Poppa Joe that "Nana won't share her markers!!!" Thing One prayed… "Nana would not have any cancerohhhs". I love these girls!!

Sept. 30th 2013 (by Wes Weber)

A couple days ago our world was turned upside down when we found out that Mom had cancer. The outpour of support has been amazing, as several of you have contacted us to let us know that we were in your thoughts and prayers. Many of you know Mom. Some of you may just know Dad or one of us boys. We appreciate y'all and the support you have shown us. We have created this site to keep everybody informed of Mom's progress, and as a place for all to turn to for encouragement, especially those who are fighting cancer, or other devastating health issues

Chapter 2

Hopping on the Roller Coaster

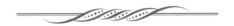

Well... it was a busy day and I hardly know where to start. First off, let me just say....I really like the doctor who is going to be my surgeon. He is a Christian and when I told him we have people from 32 states and 2 other countries praying for us, he said..."Have them pray for me too!" He told me he wouldn't do anything to compromise my health.

It looks like there is going to be a bit of change in plans. Because the tumors are 2 and 4 centimeters, I am going to have to have chemo for about 4 months before surgery. I will have a small surgery next week to put a port in for the chemo. If I get over this cough I have, then chemo will start in about two weeks. I will have a mastectomy. He said my care is going to start moving very fast.

YES... I am a wimp! There I said it. You know it I know it. Everybody knows it now, but we're going to whip this thing. I may need a lot of hand holding but a girl doesn't have to like losing her hair!!! My son Wes Weber told me he's going to shave his head too. Those who know him know that's funny.

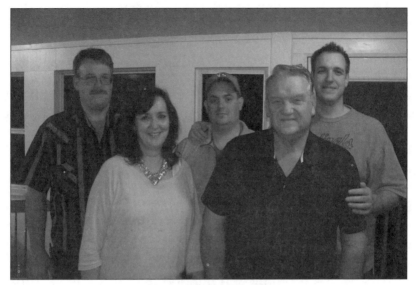

**My beautiful family!
Timothy, Wes and James
Me and my wonderful husband!**

October 6th, 2013

I wanted to thank everyone for continuing to pray for me (& my family). I have been overwhelmed at the support and prayers that have gone up for me. Earlier we asked everyone to list their state. I was overwhelmed to hear from thirty five states and four different countries. I am so blessed! I'm praying for you too!!! I mean that!!!

Thank you God...for our blessings today!

October 7th, 2013

I am going Friday a.m. to see when I will get my port put in. Pray that this thing will SHRINK and not spread!   FEAR be GONE in Jesus name!

October 9th, 2013

I had a little come apart, pity party today. Nobody showed up but me so that wasn't much fun! Really silly after having had such a wonderful ladies night out last night at church and hearing the testimonies of how hard some of them are having it in other countries. Silly me!

October 10th, 2013

I spent today with some of my very favorite people!! Thing One and Thing Two and my parents! Thing One turned FIVE years old today and she told everyone who came within hearing distance!! What a joy it was to be with her!! Yesterday when I took her back to her mommy she hugged my neck several times and said..."Nana...I'm praying for you!" How precious is that!!

Tomorrow is a big day for me. I visit with my oncologist. I understand this is an extensive visit where they will explain my treatment and schedule me to get my port put in. I am very visual so I'm hoping I don't freak out when I see the equipment. Anybody else out there afraid of medical equipment?? I mean... things like needles... bigger needles...even bigger ones??? What's all of this stuff anyway? If they put a port in, does that mean my ships coming in??? Ha! Ha! Ha! Please pray that I will be calm with God's peace and that those who have my health in their care will be led by God. I covet your prayers and I'm praying for you too!!!!!

October 11th, 2013

Have you ever done something you said you would not do???

It seems like I am eating a lot of my own words!! I know I have said out loud and not just in my head... I won't take a flu shot! I wouldn't do chemo! I'm not letting anyone cut on ME!!! BAM! BAM! BAM! Forget that!

Today I got a flu shot. Joe got one too so he wouldn't take a chance of being sick around me. Even Thing One got one at her Five year old checkup today! Afterwards we got together and compared band aids!! She got a purple one with designs on it. I got a plain brown one. Thing One still bragged on it for me and thought it was nice! I thought her purple one was cool! The things you can do when you have "friend support!"

Well... we are still at the hurry up and wait part of my treatments. I have to meet with a genetic counselor next week and have a PET scan done to see if cancer is showing up any place else. We are waiting on the doctor to schedule surgery to put the port in and to remove sentinel nodes. All new big words.

We visited the chemo room. It wasn't as scary as it sounds. I think they heard I was coming and hid all the knives and needles and wires and things and brought out fruit, candy and snacks!

I did find out that I cannot use the ICE CAP as way too often when women use it, they don't lose their hair BUT it prevents the chemo from doing its job and way too often the cancer returns. So.... I guess... bald it is and we'll face that when we face it!

It's disappointing that during chemo... I won't be able to shake hands or hug. I'm both a shaker and a hugger! But I CAN take Face book hugs!!! I feel like I'm taking nursing school or something. I'm learning so much! Your prayers were felt today! Thank you! Even if I don't answer your post individually (due to time and being overwhelmed) I do see them all and appreciate them AND I'm praying for you too!!!

October 16th, 2013

Things are starting to roll. Thursday genetic counseling. Friday "Echo" test. Wednesday, PET scan. I do believe I've been at the doctor's office more this past month than I have in five - ten years!

October 17th, 2013

I lost my cousin to lung cancer yesterday. I'm going to miss you Steve Adams! Steve was a little over a year younger than me!

RIP Steve!

October 18th, 2013

Happy, happy, happy... weepy, weepy, weepy. Happy, happy, weepy, weepy. I'm sure glad for naps to help us change our mood!!

Today was a busy day. I had my ECHO gram today. I'm wondering if that's a little bit like a singing gram that keeps repeating its self. It seems like it, since they suggested I may have to have one every three months. Anyway, as far as we can tell, I have a good heart! I had another doctor appointment and it looks like (& I say this tongue in cheek since so many things have changed on me) next Tuesday, I get my port in and lymph node surgery to see if the cancer has spread to any nodes. (Praying it hasn't) On Wed, I have my PET scan. I don't even have a pet! Maybe I'll take the neighbor's cat since he's adopted US!! Chemo starts the next week and I'll have it every other week. I got my pneumonia shot today. Thank you for your prayers! I pray God blesses you abundantly! He can do that you know!!

October 21st, 2013

Happy 80th Birthday to my sweet little mommy who is still 39!!

I have to be at the hospital at 10 a.m. for the port tomorrow. Thank you for your prayers. Please pray for my little mommy as this is very hard on her! Thank you all! Even those who are strangers to me but know my sons or are a friend of a friend! I notice you and appreciate your prayers. You're all the best!! I praise God for my support team!!!

Good news!!! I got my test results back today and I do not have the bad HR2 (whatever that is) and I won't have to take the extra two other chemo on top of my regular chemo!!! Praise God for HIS goodness!!

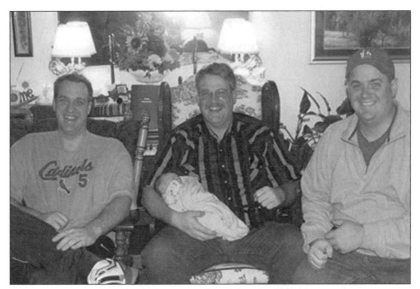

LIFE IS BRIGHT….. I have three sons!!!
James, Timothy and Wesley

October 23rd, 2013

I really think there are places that should never have a needle put in them, but that's beside the point. I faced the fear of surgery yesterday and passed with flying colors! The sentinel node test was something else though. No thank you sir! Today I'm SORE. I'm getting ready to go get my PET scan. Butterscotch must know it's today as he hasn't come around this morning.

    Thank you to all who came to the hospital to see me! Your smiling faces and positive attitudes mean so much! Thank you to my dear mom and dad who came and spent the night with us last night and thank you to my sweet darling hubby who spoiled me just a little bit more!!! I'm praying today as I go thru the PET scan that the cancer has not spread to any other location!!! I'm praying for you too!!!

October 25th, 2013

Nodes are CLEAR!! Wahoo! Yeah!! Yippy! Yippy!! Rah! Rah! Rah! CHEERS! I am so EXCITED!!! Thank you for hearing our prayers Lord!!! Thank you friends and family for praying!!!
    Chemo training was "over whelming" today. I hope I can remember everything. I just remember they don't want me to throw up!! Hum! I don't want to throw up either! That's funny! Chemo starts Tuesday and goes every other week for 4 aggressive rounds. Surgery, and then 12 more weeks of once a week chemo. They also told me I will be tired! UGH! I hate being tired!!! Now that all my tests are underway, we're ready to get this thing rolling and shrink BOO BRAT right outta here!!! Thanks for hanging in there with me!! I love you each and am praying every day for YOU!!!

October 28th, 2013

I can always be encouraged when I come to my face book page (Karen's Cancer Kickin Crew)! Thank you Wes Weber for setting it up for me! I love you boys so much!!! I'm not sure I'll have time to check in here in the morning as it is DAY ONE of CHEMO. I'm totally nervous and I hope I don't embarrass myself when they stick that chemo in my port. I am determined that my verse will be... "This is the day the Lord has made...I will rejoice and be glad in it!" I am told that once I have my first treatment that the cancer will cease to grow!! Wahoo!!! Thank you my friends for taking this journey with me!!! Thank you to my sister-in-law (Theresa Robinett) who is a breast cancer survivor of 14 years who has come to be with me for a few weeks. I'll be praying for you too!! You can count on it!

October 29th, 2013 (Dad's 83rd birthday) First day of Chemo!!!!!!!

Thing One was so concerned about Nana losing her hair and looking like a boy! I showed her a wig. I wish I had a picture of her face as she'd never seen a wig before. She got to try it on and play around so I think we're a little more prepared for that big step!

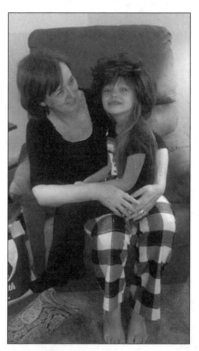

Yes! I took my apple to Chemo with me!!! My apple that reminds me that "I am the apple of God's eye"!

Chapter 3

Hair Today, Gone Tomorrow

November 1st, 2013

As one who eats dark chocolate and drinks COKE or DR Pepper for any kind of ailment... I've been a little loopy with all the items being deposited in my "scared to death of medication body".

That being said, excuse the loopy and continue on this journey with me. I woke up "chemo day" weepy; feeling like I was really facing a giant head on. NOT the "This is the day the Lord has made... I will rejoice in it" day that I had planned. After a few tears the Lord gave me my morning verse..."I can do all this through him who gives me strength" Philippians 4 v 13. Not only did I need YOUR prayers, but I needed to know MINE counted too!!

I jumped all the hoops with Joe and Theresa (my s-i-l) and my sister Jill by my side. My first exciting news was that I was downgraded from Stage IIIB to Stage IIB AND instead of cancer being in all three nodes that they took, it's just in ONE!! Praise God!!

After that excitement I went back to the Chemo room to see where my dear friend Claudia had a surprise tea-party with real china and cloth napkins, cookies, lemon slices all spread out for me!!! You KNOW I love being spoiled! With Jill's "Sister Book" and my tea-party and good news, it helped erase the frost bite spray for the port (that made me lose my pride) time earlier!

My nurse navigator (Carol Walters) brought out some wigs and caps for me to look at. We laughed and goofed around with them. I can't imagine myself without my long hair so the feelings are really going over my head. Will I REALLY lose my hair? Surely not!

Time to inject the dreaded medication. They gave me a little something to settle nerves, plugged me in and I promptly fell asleep! Oh happy, happy, me! Oh loopy, loopy me!

I'm so thankful for my support group (which includes every one of you too!!!) It has meant so much to me! I grew lazy for a couple of days at mom and dad's house. I am back home now waiting for the next step.

My song came later in the day, and it continues..."This is the day the Lord has made; I will rejoice and be glad in it"! I woke this morning feeling good at 4 a.m. (you KNOW that isn't me!) so I started praying for you all; as many as I could remember name by name. You mean so much to me! Even those of you who are strangers by name but not by heart!!! Thank you for remembering me! It humbles me!! Oh yeah... I still have my hair!!!

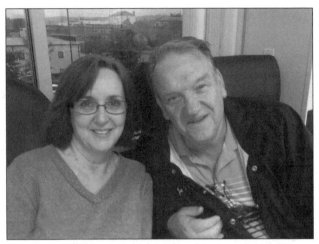

Karen & Joe 1st day of chemo!

November 2nd, 2013

I could hardly believe I'd be so lazy in one day or my mind in such a fog, but that's how yesterday went. Our first day of having Thing One and Thing Two at the house in two weeks! I mentioned I was a bit "shaky" and Thing One told me..."Oh Nana! I'll be your walking stick!" This has really been hard on her tender little heart! Today Thing Two turns THREE YEARS OLD!!

November 3rd, 2013

Thank you God for Sunday! A day of rest. A day of worship. A new start to the week. Watch out Monday... Here I come ready for you!!!!!

November 5th, 2013

Thank you my friends and family who are standing in the gap for me! I love you each and every one!!! Does anybody know what today is????

November 7th, 2013

Thank you God for good days and that melt downs don't really count anyway!!!

November 8th, 2013

Today....I am thankful for Thing One and Thing Two! Two excited little girls bounced into our house today!!! Thing One drew a picture of the two of us. Her with hair. Nana with breast cancer! We had long skinny legs and feet that looked like chicken feet! Not a lot of anything else but smiles and standing close!!!

Thing Two brought me her picture. I held the scribbles up and said, "Now... what did YOU draw?" Her face had a stunned look on it and she said, "Oh I missed a spot!!!" Then she drew a green circle, poked a hole in it and looked at me thru it! I said, "I see a big blue eye!!" Still looking back thru the hole, she said to me, "I see a big brown eye!" Oh the fun we had today with Thing One and Thing Two in the house!!! When they left... Thing One was crying so hard. She looked up at me with tears in her eyes and said, "Is there something of yours I can just carry with me?" Yep, I bawled too. Thank you God for these two precious granddaughters you've blessed us with.

November 9th, 2013

Actually I was giggling as I did it!!! For the past three weeks since my first surgery; I have not been by myself!!! I must say, I am truly THANKFUL for my family and especially for my precious sister-in-law Teresa who came to spend these first few weeks to help me get started on my journey. She and Joe went to town for a couple of things a bit ago. I grabbed my bucket, squeegee and paper towels and got the bay windows done!!! They are sparkling!!! Tee Hee!!! Go me!!!!

November 11th, 2013

It seems like whenever something big or exciting is going to happen; I just can't sleep. I sneak out of bed (after tossing an hour) and head to my journal. That verse in I Corinthians 11 keeps running thru my mind. "If a woman has long hair, it is her glory".

I run my fingers thru my short hair, I've always had hair! When I was a little girl I wore pigtails with ribbons on the ends of them. In high school my hair was at my waist. I learned early on a girl can swing her hair to match her attitude! I've had it long. I've had it short. I've worn it up. I've worn it down. I've donated it to Locks of Love. I've worn pigtails and pony tails. But I've never, ever NOT had hair! Truth be told...I can't even imagine it!

I keep running my fingers thru my hair, over and over and I still cannot comprehend it in my mind that within the week it's supposed to be gone. Chemo Two...Tuesday morning. It's funny, I've been shown, wigs and hats and scarves and even how to make cute turbans out of tee - shirts. But I haven't put anything on my head yet.

I keep wondering.... what am I really going to do. Am I going to cry? They tell me everyone does and that it's ok. Am I going to cover the mirror and just not look? Maybe. Am I going to dance for Jesus and plead "just help me thru this"??? Or am I going to crawl under the blankets and not come out for a week??? I don't know, but Thing One and Thing Two will be in the house tomorrow. I think we're going to go hat shopping and buy us three girls each a new hat!!! In the meantime, THANK YOU for praying for me and know I'm still praying for YOU! I'm thankful for hair today!

Oh my goodness.....I did not expect all of the responses I got on my post early this morning!!! Thank you for sharing your heart with me!!! I laughed and giggled and cried with you! I just want each of you to know that I feel the peace of your prayers!!! Thank you for walking this journey with me!!!

I had a fabulous day today!! Thing One and Thing Two were in the house before I was out of bed this morning!! What a way to wake up!!! We were piled up (all three of us) in my recliner like we are so often and I announced that we were going "Hat shopping" today for all three of us!! They out voted me!!! They said they already have a hat and "mommy is making you a hat, but it's a secret and you (that would be me!) can't know about it". They continued, "We don't need to go hat shopping, we just want to stay at your house all day!

I couldn't let that pass now...could I???? Would you??? I said, "Well now, I'll just have to wait and see what color it will be!!!" To which both girls replied in unison...."Red!! But you can't know! It's a surprise!" So....today....we had a tea party with real china, played with play dough, painted with water color, snuggled and snuggled!!! What a wonderful day! Tomorrow is Chemo 2. I'm working up my courage to be plugged in again. Today.... I am thankful that I feel like kickin' up my heels. Just keeping it real here in chemo world.

November 12th, 2013

Here we go...1st day of hair loss... 2nd chemo trip. See ya in a couple... Thank you for your prayers. I'm praying for you too!

November 14th, 2013

Tomorrow my sister-in-law goes back home. She has been here with us on our first three weeks of this journey. What a wonderful sister! She has rubbed my back as I cried, sat by me during chemo, encouraged me every step of the way. Cheered me as I've pulled clumps of hair out of my head. Fixed me meals, ran my sweeper, helped with laundry, drove me places, helped me walk when I wobbled, and stayed by my side. I love her dearly. She has not once complained. She has laughed with me when I get my words and sentences backwards. We have giggled, cried, chattered and fellowshipped these three weeks. Thank you Theresa for selflessly giving us these three weeks. Thank you God for giving us Theresa!!!

I love days when we get to have Thing One and Thing Two around! Yesterday was one of those days. When we were taking them home, Thing One started in on her favorite "in the car game". She said, "I spy with my little eye something PINK!" Thing Two replied, "Is it that BLUE car???" Oh how I love those girls!

Thinking of my cousin Steve who passed last month with cancer. Today would have been his birthday! Missing you Steve!

November 16th, 2013

Today.... I am thankful for the mail lady. For the many beautiful, funny, encouraging cards, notes and letters I have received. One of those cards was from a young friend of mine. (Tatumn Bailey) She goes past my house almost every day on her way to and from work. She told me that when she goes past my house she starts praying for me! How SWEET is that!

Today my parents came and stayed with me while hubby worked. Mom made me some potato soup! The best ever and cornbread! My little mommy is 80 years old. I feel like I need to be waiting on her instead of her trying to wait on me.

I read the post from yesterday. I must be the luckiest girl ever! I know I have the best friends in the whole world and I do appreciate your encouragement! I don't have as much hair today as yesterday, but that's ok. Your encouragement has helped me more than you know. What's hair anyway but something that seems to shed all over the place.

This morning I leaned over the tub and washed what little bit of hair I had left. It began to fall out in huge clumps and reminded me of hairy little black mice floating in the water. Every place I washed a handful fell out. I have never felt as devastated in my life as I looked at my hands full of hair. I wept and I wept as I buckled over with a towel drying my bald head. That precious guy of mine just took my comb and fixed the fuzz that was left, kissed my bald head, then held me in his arms as I continued to sob. How sweet is that!!!

November 17th, 2013

I was up this morning....4 a.m. studying and having quiet time. Thinking of and praying for all of you. I was so excited that I was going to get to go to church. But... alas... when the time to go rolled around; I just wasn't able to go. It was a good day however; my sister and her husband came this afternoon for a visit. Joe made me a roast with potatoes and carrots!! A couple phone calls. "This is the day the Lord has made...I will rejoice and be glad in it!" Thank you Lord for today! I loved listening to my Christian music this morning. What a good lift for the day!

November 18th, 2013

Things I have observed today... You can sleep all night and still want to sleep all day! It's encouraging to see people at the doctor's office as they go thru their procedures and are feeling better! You can talk with strangers and be encouraged! People really do care! There's a lot of people out there with hair on their head! There's a lot of people wearing hats! If people built their homes nearer the road...it wouldn't be so far to walk to the front door. It would be nice if there were parking spots for chemo patients! A nap in the middle of the day can change your attitude. Thank you Thing One for insisting day care prayed for your Nana today!

Oh my goodness...Joe just informed me that we will be married 38 years this Friday! What to do...what to do...

November 21st, 2013

Yeah! I'm finally feeling better today! I haven't been able to get on here because 1. I didn't feel like walking down the hall to my office. 2. My computer and I had a big fight! Joe has loaned me his laptop! Yeah Joe! My baby sister took a day of vacation and came and helped me. She packed up all of my summer clothes and got my winter clothes out! Not just anyone can do a job like that for you!!! Thank you Jill for the great, great day!

Yesterday we got to have Thing One and Thing Two for the day and three of my friends came and brought me a lunch! Feeling blessed!

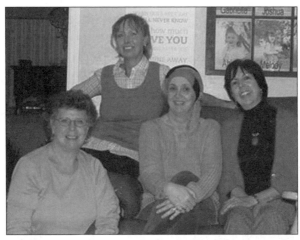

**Thank you my friends, for such an uplifting day!
(Loretta Phelps, Marsha Snodgrass & Christine Richards)
Thank you LaVern Conley for my beautiful scarves!!!**

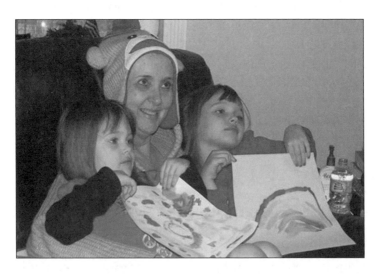

    I was afraid Thing One and Thing Two would be afraid of me with most of my hair gone and just twigs left... but no...They walked right in, climbed on my lap and put their hats on my head! (Which I had to wear all day!) They even painted pictures for me!!! Love these girls!

November 22nd, 2013

Happy 38th anniversary to Joe and me! Thirty Eight wonderful beautiful years! We celebrated by eating quarter pounders from McDonalds (just like we had on the drive the day we married). We took out our love letters we'd written while courting and read them to each other. We laughed and laughed at how "mushy" they were! (We're still pretty mushy!)

Thirty Eight years ago, Joe knocked the "Miss" from in front of my name and I became "Mrs." A title I have loved and worn proudly. Here are some random facts about us.

1. We started dating the end of September 1975
2. Joe proposed to me on October 18th, 1975
3. We were married November 22, 1975
4. We met in April 1975 briefly at a church meeting and did not see each other again until July (briefly) again at his grandparents' house for a get together. Then we did not see one another until Labor Day weekend. Hum... I think that's about three times.
5. Joe's cousin Sherry Hamilton has been my best friend for 38 years. She was our match maker. He's been my cowboy (He used to always wear boots and a hat) and I've been "his girl" ever since.
6. When we married, Joe had not met my parents or immediate family. He met my mother about a month later and my dad six months later! Yes, they were concerned!
7. We have three wonderful sons and six perfect grandchildren!
8. We owned a lumber business for more years than I can count. Now Joe teaches law enforcement and I train people on getting toxins out of their homes.
9. Joe got a head injury the year our second child was born and we (yes we) struggled with this injury for years.

Goodbye cowboy hat! All of our kids were surprises! Having all boys was even a bigger surprise!
10. Joe has lost both of his parents and I count his sisters as my own!
11. I still have both of my parents (80 and 83) and Joe says my sister is a #10
12. We have never stopped being best friends and laugh at/with each other all the time!
13. We still hold hands! We still smile at each other! We still sit close!
14. We can talk for hours to each other. We've never stopped dreaming!
15. We have traveled extensively and are happy to stay home. (or go)
16. If we eat out, you will not find the same items on our plates. Most of our taste in anything is as different as daylight and dark.
17. We have lots of secrets about us! We'll never tell.... aw come on!
18. Our first meal after we got married was at McDonalds in Columbia on our way to Kansas City. Joe introduced me to the new quarter pounder! We still like to celebrate with a quarter pounder.
19. Joe's sisters told me (on the day that we were married) that Joe would not eat anything except hamburger. After about three months, Joe got up the nerve to ask me if I could come up with something different. Boy was I happy when I found out they'd been teasing me! You'd be surprised at what all I can do with hamburger!
20. I literally burnt our first meal the day after we were married. I mean, the oven was literally in flames! We received many gifts at our wedding and probably every appliance available except a toaster. I fixed toast in the oven and because SOMEBODY distracted me it burnt to a crisp. We literally had to put the fire out! Joe laughed and I cried! It was all of the bread we had so

we ended up having crackers with our eggs. Yep, we still have that once in a while just to remember!

Since we are at another thru sickness and health part of our marriage this year we have decided to have quarter pounders from McDonalds today. We dug out the letters we wrote (yep... we wrote letters every day) for the month and a half that we dated and read them to each other. It's going to be another great, great day with my "Mr."

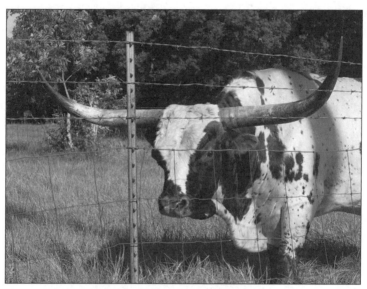

**The "Bull" became the
symbol of my chemo treatments and shots!**

November 24th, 2013

Joe and I were {both} excited to get to go to church this morning! It proved to be worth the effort of getting out of bed and out of the house! We love our church body and our pastor and his wife. We came home and I promptly slept away the afternoon.

Now I'm thinking about this coming week. Chemo is...I think maybe a little bit like riding a bull. I've never had the desire to ride a bull. In fact, I watch bull riding thru my fingers. Things get tough and I close my eyes!

I'm working up my courage to go back and get on the bull again this Tuesday. I don't look when they give me a shot. I don't look when they "plug me in". I've never looked at the "plug in". Instead, I close my eyes. When they've got me all plugged in and going, I look around the room at the many people there; going thru what I'm going thru.

Oddly enough, there seems to be more men in the room than women. I wonder about everyone's story! What kind of cancer do they have? How are they handling it? Do they have a great support team like I do? Often our eyes meet in recognition and we share a smile. Silent support! The "we can do this" look that we all share! We all know it's going to be a rough week; that chemo, not turkey is what's going to make most of us sleepy on Thursday. We're so thankful for those supporting us with their prayers. Remember....we are praying for you too!!!

Thing One (5).... "Nana...you might not have hair...but I still love you!"

Thing Two (3)...."Nana is beautiful!" (Honest! I didn't coach them!)

November 26th, 2013

I was pretty weepy today before they put the quarters in that bull I had to ride. I had a good doctor visit and hope this time, with some medication I will be able to bypass a bit of the pain around my port and heart area as I ride the bull this week. DR Nevils is also pretty sure my surgeon is going to schedule my surgery in December after my next chemo treatment. My tumors have decreased significantly! So all is on schedule and looking good.

That being said...Thank you to my sister Jill and my nurse navigator Carol Walters for supporting me this morning and helping me thru the rough spots! Also thanks to DR Nevil's, nurses Juli Terry and Stephanie Pritchett for all of their support!!! A special thanks for my Joe! All of you know how to turn tears to smiles!! I love each of you!

Thing Two (3) was here yesterday. I laid down with her to try to get her to take her nap. As you do with a little one, you pretend you are asleep! I closed my eyes. She looked me over real good and then started rubbing my almost completely bald head over and over. Over and over....over and over. (Like she was petting me.) Then she petted my face, kept patting my head and put her little forehead against mine and gave me an Eskimo kiss. Then she kissed my face. She put her arm around my neck and laid there but she never did go to sleep!!! My heart smiled!

November 27th, 2013

Well I rode that bull with one hand in the air yesterday and I did it again today! After I got over my weepy dread time; I did great!! Yeah! Go me!

Our middle son came home from Topeka last night and got in around midnight. Even though we knew we shouldn't; he and I sat up and talked until around 3 a.m. this morning! Wes is the one who set up my web site for us! He attends Washburn Law School.

I was telling him about how lazy I've been feeling. It's really kind of funny. Last spring while I was mentoring a bible study class; I was kind of feeling this lazy feeling coming on. Now for those who know me... I'm not lazy. I like to accomplish things and get things done. Put me under pressure and I can do miracles. However... I kept having this worry, I'm feeling like I could be lazy and enjoy it. I'd asked for prayer against wanting to be lazy.

Now several months later, I'm spending hours in my recliner. I can look at the sweeper and think.... I need to run the sweeper....check... I thought about it! That's as far as my energy goes. About the only thing I've been consistent with is making the bed! I hate an unmade bed!!! I need to dust...

check... I thought about it! You get the picture! So back to our conversation....

Wes asked me if I'd ever heard of the "Mary fight". No.... "How about the Mary fight, Martha fight"? Ah now...that makes sense. My Mary and Martha personalities certainly aren't balanced!!! I rather enjoy being Martha!!!

Wes looked me straight in the eye and said "If you don't hear anything else that I say to you tonight, hear this! You might want to write it down!" "Today....I'm going to be Mary!" So, the dust can accumulate, the dishes can wait, the dust on the ceiling fans can wait, the sweeper can wait, the bathroom cleaning can wait, the kitchen floor can wait to be mopped, the laundry can wait!

Today....I'm going to be Mary. I'm going to sit at HIS feet and learn whatever is it I'm supposed to learn during this time in my recliner. What is God's purpose for me for the remainder of my life? If I can let Mary win the fight...the last half of my life can be far richer than the first half of my life. Thank you God for a wise son that you are sharing with me. Thank you for speaking to me through my son! I love you Lord and don't want to disappoint you!

November 29th, 2013

I certainly hope I don't offend with my post today. It's not my intention. The other night I woke up in the middle of my slumber. As you know...when I wake up, I love to pray for you. Seeing how many names I can remember and bringing you and yours before a caring God. It's my thank you to you for all of your support and prayers. Well, this particular morning, I couldn't think of one name...not one. "God... why can't I think of one name?" Immediately the thought came to me..."I didn't wake you up to pray; I woke you up to listen to ME!" Ah here goes the Mary/Martha fight already!

I didn't get the wish I wanted at the doctor the other day. My tumors have shrunk, very much, excitedly so!!! But still the doctor says I will lose everything on my left side! Needless to say, I'm not happy about that! I've thought of those verses in the bible that says..."If your hand offends you... cut it off..."etc. hum!

I don't think I've ever used my body in a way to offend. I've tried not to. If I have...I'm sorry. I can understand more if part of my mind had to go but I'm grateful, I'm getting to keep my brain! So why am I having to have part of me cut off??? Why Lord...why???

I'm right handed. That means I've cuddled my three sons in my left arm. I cuddle Thing One and Thing Two with hugs on my left arm. I've held each one close to my chest. When I say the pledge, I put my hand over my left side. Now...there's going to be nothing! NOTHING at all??? Why not the other side?? Why Lord?? Now there will just be a scar! Oh... I get it! You want me to remember the scars on YOUR body. What you went thru for ME! You want me to remember more vividly and GROW! When I place my hand on my chest, there will be no fluff...just a scar. There will be no fluff between my hand and my heart! I'll be thinking..."I pledge allegiance to God!" Lord... grow me gently! Please be easy! I'm a wimp, and I'm scared.

November 30th, 2013

I wish I could answer each one of your posts individually. You are each such an encouragement to me. I seriously don't feel I need to be bragged on or told how good I'm doing. Seriously...I'm just sitting here in this ole comfy recliner in my jammies. I've not accomplished anything yet! My house isn't as clean as it could be. I sleep a lot.

Today I wasn't able to help Joe and the boys decorate the porch for Christmas. I was really looking forward to that. Still, they did an awesome job without me. Now I need to take the pumpkins down from inside and get out some cheery snowmen. I thought about it… check! I have so much to be thankful for! There's nothing like having a son walk in and give you a kiss on your almost bald head! The love of my family and friends amaze me! Today I got to take my list out of all of your names here and pray for each of you. Some of you are going thru some challenging times! You are not forgotten!

Thank you to my wonderful sons Wes and James for coming and hanging a little Christmas cheer on our front porch! I love you guys so much!!!!

Chapter 4

Bull Riding Gone Wild

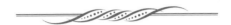

December 1st, 2013

I so wanted to be able for church this morning!

It sure was hard to say goodbye to my sons as they head back to Washburn Law School. Thanks for the hugs, decorating, lemon donuts and most of all for the visiting!! I love you guys and hope you ace those finals coming up!! Can't wait to see you again!

December 2nd, 2013

Three days of hard bull riding. I am going to "whup" that bull! Might need a new pair of spurs... but I'm going to do it!!

December 3rd, 2013

I rode the bull today and he threw me off. I ended up having to get IV's and prescriptions. On the upside... I've lost some weight! (Enough to count) I got to see Thing One and Thing Two today. I lost count of how many times they said..."I love you Nana!" Gonna ask Santa for some diamond studded spurs. I've got to let that bull know whose boss!!!

December 4th, 2013

Thank you Karen Stephens for coming and putting our Christmas tree up for us today!!! How cheerful!!!! So appreciated your help and the homemade noodle soup!

Thank you to my baby sister for coming and cleaning for me and spreading Christmas cheer over our house! Thank you for taking the pumpkins down! Love you to the moon and back!

December 5th, 2013

Sometimes I wonder about the lady whose been sitting in my chair! It's like she's taken it and won't move! She's not like me at all! I like to get 'er done!

I wouldn't consider myself a Diva, though I've been accused of it enough times. I'm an eastern gal born and raised in the Buckeye state. I like to dress up, I like it to match. I like colors, bold and action. I use the #7 rule when dressing. I don't even mind if I shock you once in a while. I once teased Pastor Dave that he could preach on vanity all he wanted but I was still going to have my jewelry matching even if it made me late! I don't think he was preaching at me anyway. He never does! Bahahhahaha! It may not be in place when I get there, but it was when I left!

The other day I was walking past the full length mirror thru our bedroom when I saw my reflection. I actually did a two-step backwards and said "Who in the world is that!" I thought someone else had moved in. It's that lady who's always stealing my chair! There she was looking like an ostrich with big black circles under her eyes and oh I had to laugh at her hair, or lack thereof! There's just "scraglies" left.

On this particular day, the static electricity had it standing straight up! How can you not have hair and still need a haircut is beyond me! You would have laughed too! I'm pretty comfortable with my hair gone now. It's not a pretty site but the lady in the chair is ok with it. I'm just anxious to get some energy.

There's so many things I want to do. But I'm happy and that's a fact a jack!

December 7th, 2013

I am so missing Christmas shopping, baking cookies and candy this year!!! I'm missing going to the craft shows and the parties. I'm missing flying saucer riding and snowball fighting. I'm missing Thing One and Thing Two!!!! Missing my sister and our annual Christmas shopping day. Missing shopping with friends and eating out!! Missing the jing jing jingling of the season.

December 8th, 2013

I got to be me today!!! I did two loads of laundry, made a bunch of little gift bags and worked on Christmas Cards. Joe and I watched a Beth Moore bible study this morning. My Christmas shopping is done. Everything done from right here in my home except when Joe went to the store for us!

Our tree is up. It looks beautiful even though we are not going to put any ornaments on it this year. It has berries and cones and is pre-lit so it's beautiful on its own. We'll miss putting the ornaments on because each one has its own story and is from places we have traveled. It's always fun to take them out and remember but we're not going anywhere this year so we're going to skip the decorations and that's ok!

I'm trying to get up the courage to get back on the bull Tuesday. That bull still scares me spitless and I dread how I feel afterwards but this is the last one until surgery. I'm praying that my blood count is up enough for this last treatment and that I will shed this cough.

The bible study we watched this morning was on Joshua 1 and how many times God had to tell this strong warrior to be brave and that He would go before him. Over and over HE told him to be brave and courageous. Go away fears! Be gone!!! I'm still praying for you all. It has become one of my favorite things to do as I remember your faces and names. Even if I don't know you personally, you are still on my list!!! I appreciate your support and encouragement and most of all your prayers!

December 9th, 2013

GO AWAY fever!!! I AM getting on that bull tomorrow!! I did some more laundry today! Surely I haven't developed a reaction to doing laundry!! Joe took Thing One and Thing Two shopping today. He now believes he is superman! I'm not sure they got any shopping done but I know there was an incident about somebody not wanting to ride in the buggy and somebody else wanting to ride on the front where she could drag her shoe! Please pray that my fever will go away, and that this terrible cough goes away. I can hardly talk without coughing. I really need to finish up this round of Chemo tomorrow; much as I dread it. Thank you and I will continue to pray for YOU!

December 10th, 2013

I went by today and kicked the bull. Somehow I just couldn't help but taunt him a little. But... I didn't get on him even though he was saddled up and I was plugged in. After waiting for the blood work to come in, my doctor was afraid I would end up in the hospital if I rode the bull today. So we unsaddled and headed home to try and build myself up a bit this week.

Looks like this will likely change surgery date. We won't know for a bit. My fever did go away and my cough is better. Thank you for your prayers!!!

Want to hear a knee slappin' funny? When you take chemo, you get something they call "chemo brain". It works like this... sometimes you can't think straight and can't get your words out right. I've had a difficult time spelling. One day I even had to ask Joe how to spell Thing One's name!! I know, crazy huh!

Well, I wanted to tell Joe that we needed to add water to the air because the air was too dry for me and it was hurting my nose. I wanted to explain that I no longer have nose hairs.

That's funny in itself! How it KEPT coming out was that I no longer have hose nairs! I could not get it right! Yep, there's your knee slapper for the day!

December 11th, 2013

Surgery date has been changed from Dec 30th to January 7th, 2014

December 13th, 2013

I really need to get over this cough. My port area has swollen and I need for the swelling to go down. I have to be ready to get back on the bull Tuesday. I think if I could quit the coughing maybe the swelling would go down. I was able to fix supper tonight. Left overs in the microwave. Thanks Barb Sanders for bringing us supper last night. Yum Yum! Thanks Mom and Dad for sitting with me while Joe worked. Thanks Sarah Parks for such a special visit! Thank you all for praying for me

December 14th, 2013

I've been writing Merry Christmas and I hope your family has the BEST 2014 Happy New Year ever on several cards. I've been thinking about 2013 and getting this year wrapped up. It was a good year until... but you all know THAT story!
    I got to travel with Joe some. I enjoyed watching Thing One and Thing Two. Sometimes five days a week! We had so much fun! The hugs and cuddles, watching them grow, laughing at all the funny things they said and did. We got to do some remodeling and had plans for more. Oh how fun to see the improvements. I loved working and growing my Melaleuca business. I loved having parties and shopping with friends.
    Then one day, that all stopped. I was no longer able to travel with Joe. I wasn't even able to go with him to get groceries this morning. I miss grocery shopping. I love grocery shopping! I'm not able to watch Thing One and Thing Two. I

think I've had them a total of 3 or 4 days since chemo started. I miss them and they miss me!

The remodeling has come to a stop. I'm still dreaming though! I can't wait to get back to working on my business. I love sharing ways with others on how to get the cancer causing toxins out of their homes. I am thankful that I've been very careful about that and that my cancer isn't a toxic driven cancer.

Since September my focus has changed on everything. Now... I'm just thankful! Thankful I'm alive, thankful for my family, my friends, for wonderful doctors and nurses! I'm thankful for helping hands, and meals dropped off. For those who have run the sweeper for me. I'm thankful for prayers and for strangers praying for me. I'm thankful we bought these nice comfortable recliners early this year! I'm thankful for Joe's work team! I'm especially thankful for a husband who hasn't grown tired or weary of taking care of me. Most of all I am thankful for GOD!

I know I came into 2013 one person and will go into 2014 even another person. I'm not always sure I recognize who I am now. Sometimes I'm cheery, sometimes I'm weepy. Sometimes I'm chatty, other times I'm just quiet.

I started thinking about this "Happy New Year" that's almost here. My DR warned me that I would be grieving for a season during 2014. I hadn't thought about that but I realize I've already started the process.

The first four or five months I'm still going to have to check in for the bull ride. I look at all of the faces of those who have ridden this bull and won! It amazes me that someone can be so low and bounce back so good! I know none of us knows who we will be going into 2014.

Life can spin on a dime, but, let's be good people! Let's do the right thing! Let's help our fellow man. Let's be respectful. Let's teach our children what's right and wrong. Let's hold each other closer and encourage one another. Let's be good Americans!!! Let's thank God for our blessings and let's share those blessings with others. I know it's a little early and I know I'll repeat it later this month... But Happy New Year Everyone! I pray it's your best ever!

December 16th, 2013

Ok... here we go! I hope that old bull forgot that I kicked him on my way out last week. I'm getting back on him tomorrow. This will be my first bull ride without Joe there holding my hand! I'm not sure who is going to be sitting on my left, but I can guarantee I'm going to be squeezing the tar out of their hand!! I just hope I know who they are! Otherwise it's going to be quite a way to get acquainted!!! Please pray my port will be easy to access without any problems! Pray I won't panic and all will go smooth. Thank you for praying for me in my need! I continue to pray for you all daily! YES! That is YOU!

December 17th, 2013

Thank you! Thank you! Thank you each and every one for your prayers! Thank you God for hearing my prayers too!! I had it friends! I had my boots and spurs on. I was feeling good! I could jump in the air and click my heels!

I think that old mean bull kind of learned a lesson when I kicked him last week. I think he was kind of afraid of me!!! I got there at 9 a.m. to get plugged in and wasn't able to actually ride the bull until after 12 noon. Here's what I think happened!!

I think the bull ran and hid and it took several to go coax him back in to me!!! Little Sissy!!! Anyway, I took candy canes to share with everyone in the chemo room. My nurse navigator passed them out for me and told everyone I was celebrating this last chemo for this stage today! You would have thought it was Christmas!

People were so excited for me and that old bull didn't know for sure what was going on so he kept hiding out! I couldn't believe the people who came up and congratulated me and cheered me on! Amazing good people! I heard story after story! It's a good thing I'm already married, otherwise I think I could have picked up the little old man sitting beside me!!! (Bald and all!)

The Pink Duck

    I left chemo after 3. We ran buy Aldies and bought a trunk load of canned goods and groceries. We went by JC Penny for a few minutes and to K-Mart to pick up a gift for the girls, since I had not seen them in so long. We stopped by James and Kira's for about 30 minutes. LOVED getting to see Thing One and Thing Two. We went by mom and dads for fried apples and biscuits, then on home where we wanted to crash; but the fire was out and we had to unload the trunk load of groceries and then the phone started ringing.

    I am so thankful for my energy today!! FIRST day in forever that I've had energy like this! My legs are wobbly but that's just funny stuff and I'm feeling fine! Thank you everyone for praying for me and staying with me on this journey! I love you each and every one and I pray for each of you!!! Lord, if you aren't going there; I'm not going there either! I need you to abide in me and circle my camp!

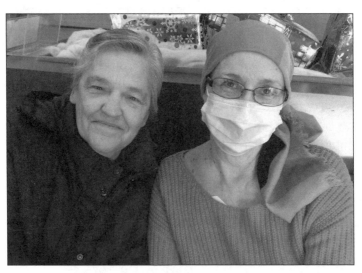

**12/17/2013 Theresa (my sis-n-law) & Karen
Last chemo before surgery.
I look like a blue duck!**

December 21st, 2013

I have to say I'm a little overwhelmed with the kindness of you all! I've been doing pretty well this week. They cut my chemo back by 10% this round and that has made a big difference in how I have felt. I was able to get out to a couple of family functions this week. Then I came home and SLEPT!

So often I hear about people who are able to work during chemo and I wonder why I'm still stuck in this chair. I guess we are all different and react to the different doses etc. Everyone's chemo is measured exactly to their situation and weight etc. My DR says that since I've not taken medication over the years that it's hitting me harder. I don't know. I just know, I so hope I feel good enough to go to Chili's and get to eat one day! That's one of my favorite places and I want to taste something that doesn't taste like chemo for once!!

I am so thankful for your prayers! The many cards and calls and visits I have received. The meals dropped off to help us out. My beautiful poinsettia from my Post Office friends! WOW! Was that not a surprise! Our website has reached hundreds of people! That is amazing! To know so many have cared and prayed for us! I am very humbled! I've been so "chemo brain" this week. But I love you each and appreciate your prayers and support. Still praying for YOU!

December 22nd, 2013

We were so excited to get to go to church this morning! The first time in several weeks! It was wonderful to get to participate in communion. Afterwards I wanted to go to Rolla for lunch. So we went to Colton's. I enjoyed my cheeseburger tremendously. Immediately afterwards I got really sick and ended up having to go by my moms. I was VERY sick until collapsing and then slept until 3; at which time Joe was able to bring me on home. I've slept most of the evening. What's with starting out so good and dropping so low? I need some "UP" days for sure!

December 23rd, 2013

I wish I could write something to inspire you but I'm not feeling too inspired. I ended up getting more IV's today. Now I'm home trying to wolf down some Imodium. That stuff is YUCK! I am so thankful for my wonderful husband who has really stood by me and done more than should be asked of any husband. The nurses and DR at the Bond Clinic are the best! I have to admire the care they give to each and every one there. Always smiling, always kind. They even shared their caramel candy with me today!

Please say a prayer for all the ones going for that last checkup to help them thru the holidays. There's some real troopers in there. Say an extra prayer for a little lady named Ruth Ann who told me today that she will have to have treatments for the rest of her life unless there is a miracle! James is bringing Thing One and Thing Two here for breakfast tomorrow! Can't wait!! Thank you for your prayers! I love you each and pray for you!

It's funny the things you remember in the middle of the night when you should be asleep! It was back in September, That awful fateful day as I sat chatting with another lady waiting on mammogram results. We were both a little weepy. Another lady came in and was waiting for her mammogram. I "sorta" apologized to her for the two of us being a little weepy. She looked at me and said..."It's just a mammogram!" I pray it was for her but it wasn't for me and I don't think it was for the lady who had just been called in. Girls! It's NOT just a mammogram! It is your LIFE!

Today I had to go for more IV's to get me back on track. It was a slow steady day at the clinic. Men and women coming and going for another checkup hoping to make it thru the holidays without having to call their DR or get sick. Everyone encouraging each other to have a Merry Christmas and to "hang in there!"

I got to wondering about this Christmas Day coming up. The day that for so many of us represent the birth of our risen

Lord! I wondered at His death and resurrection. I wondered how many said... "It's just a whipping!"? NO! It was a beating! Beyond recognition!!! Did anybody say..."It's just three days in the tomb?" NO! It was the pit of hell!! I don't know how you celebrate that! But I just want to thank my Lord for being willing to lie in that manager, for the years He walked on this earth, for His death and resurrection. For doing that for ME! Yes... I'll celebrate in any manner that I can! I will rejoice!!! I will praise your name!

Never underestimate what someone is going through or has gone through. Some are going thru financial difficulties right now. Some have no job, some don't have family. Some are going thru things alone. I have been amazed at how many have posted just this week of losing loved ones. Be kind to your family. Put past hurts in the past. Be kind to strangers. You never know what they are facing! Pay it forward!!!!! I hope you all have a VERY MERRY CHRISTMAS and find peace in your souls!

December 24th, 2013

It's a wonderful day when Thing One and Thing Two walk in the house. Thing One wants to help me and take care of me. Thing Two isn't too impressed with my hair style even though I am growing hair again. She sat on Poppa Joe's lap at the breakfast table and looked over at me with her little finger pointing at me and said... "Nana... don't cut your hair again!!!"

December 25th, 2013

There is peace in our home this Christmas Day!

December 26th, 2013

The day I was diagnosed, I already had the pizza party planned. I decided that whatever the outcome, we were going to celebrate. It was either I didn't have cancer or if I had it; they'd found it and I was going to be treated. My family was there to support me! I haven't had pizza since. That's saying a lot from this pizza lovin' girl! I like pizza! I like it home made, I like it eating out! I like it carry out! I'm ready for some pizza!!! I'm thinking maybe pepperoni and green peppers! My mom loves to order pizza in and then fix it again. She adds tons of small chopped onions and green peppers and then more cheese! mmmmmmmm I'm thinking it's time for pizza again! I just hope it doesn't taste like chemo!!!

WOW!!!! Joe went in and paid a 46 cent postage due on some papers from the hospital. Today there was 46 cents in an envelope (in our mailbox) from the post office with a note that said: "This was already taken care of!! Ho Ho Ho" This might seem like a little thing to you... but oh it touched my heart! Thank you Roger Brooks!

Thank you Dennis Schaffer for sending me a Pizza Inn Pizza!!! WOW!!! It was awesome!

December 28th, 2013

Joe was sitting there with his fore head plastered against the eye machine. DR Falkenhain kept asking... "Is this better... or worse?" Better? Worse? If you know me well... you know where my brain went!

Those words echoed from 38 years ago! For better and for worse, through richer or poorer, thru sickness and in health. I'm not sure what I thought 38 years ago but I'm pretty sure I didn't think we'd hit ALL of these in our life time OR hit some of them more than once!!

Richer... whatever that means. I'm not sure where the measuring stick starts but I've felt "richer" before. I felt richer when the bills were all paid. I've felt richer when the family was all around the kitchen table! I've felt richer when Thing One and Thing Two were both cuddled asleep on my lap and I couldn't move until they woke up. I've felt richer when I've had a quiet time and been fed again by my Lord and Savior! I've felt richer by just a squeeze of the hand and a smile from Joe. Yep... I've definitely experienced richer!

I remember once when the "for poorer" hit. The boys were little and the weather set in and shut our business down for quite some time. We had $15 and it was two weeks before Christmas. I'll never forget that year! It was the last year I didn't get our family prepared for winter way before winter started! I'm sure we've hit that "Poor" mark many times but our rich moments have far out ranked the poor.

Right now, I'm feeling richer as I look out the bay window at the beautiful red sky showing between all of the trees! It's simply beautiful!

I'm not sure we've gone thru the worse part. When you hit the better parts it tends to erase the worse parts. I know we've been blessed with many better parts!! I'm real sure our vows didn't say anything about "obey" in there! I definitely don't remember it and I wouldn't dare ask Joe about it!

Now about that thru sickness or health part... We hit that years ago when Joe sustained a head injury. He went three years without driving a car. Years under a DR care. I had sure hoped we'd done our time with that one.

Saturday mornings are one of the hardest times for me. We love to get out and about town, eat breakfast together and just have fun. It's always been our special time. I can't wait until we get that time back! Oh yeah... I like that "To have and to hold" part! That's another richer moment. I'm thanking God for those richer moments!!

December 30th, 2013

The nurse actually laughed when I gave my answer. It was a call from the hospital with a long list of questions about my health and background. Have you ever had... have you ever had.... have you ever had... You know the list: No... no... nope... no...never! It was rather a long list and my response was always the same. Have you ever... nope.

I get bored easily and it was time to shake it up a little. So when she said... "Have you ever smoked?" I answered..."Only once; in the 8th grade!"

I'm sure my lungs were saved by Mrs. Snooks that day. I absolutely loved school. I loved my teachers. I loved my classmates. I even loved learning. I loved being in JR High at Green High School, in Franklin Furnace, Ohio.

I walked a wide circle around Mrs. Snooks though. I'm not sure why. Maybe it was because she had such large brown eyes and wore glasses that made them look really big. She also wore a really wild red lipstick. She was good at giving you a stare that could stop you in your tracks! I was a little timid around her. I only remember her getting on my case twice. We won't go into the other! (But you can be sure it involved me and my same friend)

This particular day we were in Math class. The plans were already in motion. Now to get the picture right... You have to understand I was being raised a good girl in a very strict, organized Christian home. My best friend in class was Debbie Lockwood. She was wild and free. She was going to teach me how to smoke.

I think the 1st clue to Mr. Brown (our Math teacher) was... I asked to go to the bathroom. I would never have asked to leave Math class. It was my favorite class. Within two minutes, Debbie asked to leave also.

We had the bathroom window open and ready for us to climb out on the roof of the first level below if needed. I had the cigarette between my lips ready to inhale when Mrs. Snooks walked in. I didn't inhale! I totally sucked that cigarette to the bottom of my lungs!! I started coughing and turning gray. Debbie grabbed the cigarette and flushed it and tried to hide in a stall by standing on the toilet. Mrs. Snooks stood there and stared at me until I could breathe again. Then she told me to get back to class. She got Debbie out of the stall and sent her back too. Truth be known, I'm very grateful Mrs. Snooks walked in on us that day! I've never picked up a cigarette since!

December 31st, 2013

Happy New Year to all of my family and face book friends! It's been a wild year! Thank you to each of you who have encouraged me and prayed for me this year and helped me ride that bull!!! I'm not sure I could have done it without your encouragement and prayers! They have meant the world to me! My surgery is scheduled for 7:30 a.m. on January 7th. I hope 2014 will be your best year ever and that you will have peace and prosperity in your homes. I pray you and your families will be happy and healthy. Hug one another close! I never tire of praying for you!! Happy New Year!!!

CHAPTER 5

Chop! Chop! The Chopping Block!

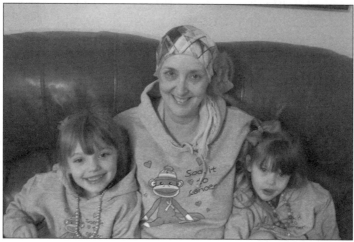

Thing One and Thing Two with Nana
Wearing our matching
"Sock it to Cancer"
Hoodies!
New Years' Day

January 1st 2014

Happy 2014 New Year Everybody! I wasn't going to but I have decided to make a New Year resolution after all. I am going to stay focused and complete the things I start. I'm always starting things and not completing them. So this year I'm going to finish everything that…

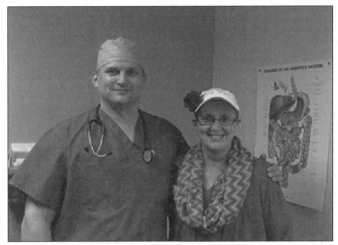

My surgeon DR Dana Voight

January 3rd, 2014

I am calmed down now...but you really wouldn't have wanted to be around me yesterday. My anger surprised even me! It blindsided me. It came out of nowhere, or so it seemed. I actually wanted to throw myself on the floor and have a two year old temper tantrum! Banging my fist and stomping my feet!!

I've been trying to take one day at a time and that's been working for me. I've been looking at my journey in three parts Chemo... Surgery.... Twelve more weeks of chemo. I've made it thru the first part. (Praise God!)

Yesterday was my last appointment with my surgeon before my surgery this Tuesday. I had to make a decision before going to the "chopping block". Am I going to "chop" or "chop... chop". For those of you on this journey with me; let me just tell you that is not an easy decision to make. It put me on an unbelievable roller coaster.

I cried all day. I cried about the beautiful sky. I cried about the snow. I cried at the lady in the mirror. I cried because I cried! I cried because I ran out of Kleenex. Nothing made sense about my crying until my nurse navigator (Carol Walters) mentioned to me that I was crying because I was grieving! That made sense, but still I cried. I cried because I was grieving! It seemed there was no thrill on the roller coaster and truth be known; I didn't know if I was going up or coming down! I've cried for what I'm putting Joe and my boys through. I cried for what I'm putting my family through. I've cried for what I'm putting Thing One and Thing Two thru and their little hearts for loving me and not understanding what's going on.

If we as adults don't understand, how can the little ones? I've cried for what I've put you my support and encouragement team through, because I know some of you will have tears reading this. I'm sorry!

I cried for the grandmother I never met who had the "chop... chop" long before I was ever born. I cried for the sister I lost to ovarian cancer. I cried because I'm scared. I cried because I missed my hair! I cried because I didn't want to be a fool and cry in front of my surgeon when I made my decision. I cried... because I didn't know what decision to make.

My surgeon (DR Dana Voight) is the best ever! He was WAY ahead of me when he walked in the room. He brought calmness and confidence. He brought everything I needed at the moment but he couldn't make the decision for me. That was still mine. The one thing I didn't want to have to make... "The decision".

I didn't want to feel guilty if I made the wrong decision. I didn't want to make a wrong decision. But I've made my decision now and I feel ok about it. I think it's the right decision for me.

Do you know if I just do the "chop" I have way over a 50%, possibly in the 60's maybe 70's chance of cancer occurring in the other side? (Because of my grandmother, my sister and the fact that I now have cancer.) That's THREE strikes!!! If I do the "chop...chop" it drops to 1%!!!!! Plus... I won't just be walking around in circles! (Ha! Ha! Now stop crying!)

Tuesday morning I will head to the "chop...chop" chopping block and grieve, I might, well... (I'm pretty sure I will), but God has given me some verses this morning. I Peter 5 verse 7 says "Cast all your anxiety on him because he cares for you." Verse

10 "And the God of all grace, who called you to his eternal glory in Christ, after you have suffered a little while, will him-self restore you and make you strong, firm and steadfast. To him be the power for ever and ever. Amen." Thank you for praying for ME! I still pray for you every day!!!

January 4th, 2014

AWESOME surprise tonight!!! Our middle son Wes (Who started Karen's Cancer Kickin Crew page for us) walked through our door!! We weren't expecting him until Sunday night or Monday!!! He called about 10 miles away and pretended he was still in Topeka!!! I LOVE those bear hugs from my boys!!!! Welcome home Wes!!!

January 5th, 2014

I don't want another day to pass without my telling YOU how much your encouragement and prayers mean to me!! On my "Oh woe is me" post the other day, I was overwhelmed with the responses between my cancer kickin' site and my personal site! Not to mention the private messages and phone calls that I received. I feel like it's only fair, if you are walking beside me on this journey that you know what's going on!

I wish I could answer each message personally! Gee... I don't even know all of you but you still reached down and helped pull me up! Amazing! I must say that the other day was by far one of my hardest days but your encouragement lifted me in a special way. Thank you!!! We are now waiting to see if our insurance will agree with my decision to go on the "chop...chop" instead of just the chopping block Tuesday. I am at complete peace with my decision!! My chemo "should" end in April (my birthday month) and I fully intend to dance in the rain to celebrate!!! So if you see me dancing... come join me!!!

January 6th, 2014

The count down to the chopping block is on! I can only eat or drink for 5 more hours and 30 minutes. That's probably the time I'll be starving and dying of thirst. Isn't that how it generally works???

Today has been a good day with my sister-in-law Theresa here and our middle son Wes. They have made sure everything is ready for me to come home. The firewood is brought in, sweeper run, floors mopped!!! I'm already looking forward to coming home! I'm not looking forward to tomorrow but am ready to have this over with.

I'm scared spitless of surgery and I don't intend to look at my scars for oh... about a year or two!!! Tonight as I lay in bed trying to fall asleep, I'm going to be praying for each of you by name. That will give me peace and we'll face tomorrow when we get there. Wes will post on here for me tomorrow after surgery sometime. Surgery is 7:30 a.m. on the dot so if you happen to be awake; think of me and say a prayer! Love you everybody!!!!!

January 7th, 2014

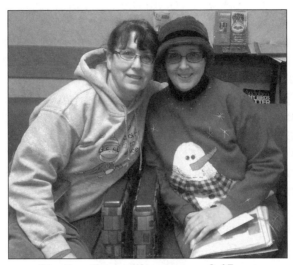

Starting the waiting game...6:15 am.
1/7/14 with my baby sister Jill.
Our sister Lynn made this sweatshirt for me before
she died of ovarian cancer.

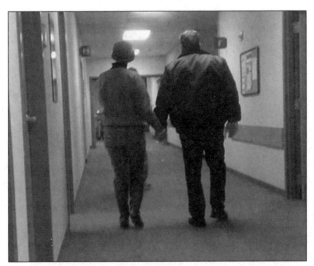

Here we go! Thanks for your prayers!!!
Heading back for surgery!!! My Joe and Me!

Just talked to the Dr. Voight. Mom is through surgery and headed for recovery. Dr. Voight said she was doing well. (By Wes Weber)

Mom told me to post for her while she was in the hospital. I didn't get to spend much time with Mom today because of a sore throat and slight temperature. Phone reception has been rather spotty so I haven't gotten many updates except that she is in her room and doing well. In spite of not getting to see her much today, there was a lesson for me that God is in control. This won't be eloquent by any means but here goes.

I had originally planned on coming home tonight to keep the fire going and to make sure that the water didn't freeze. Well I got home and you guessed it. No water. None. Now I had left the water running when we left, but in my hurry to get inside and get comfortable I completely missed the fact that the faucet wasn't running. No big deal. It shouldn't take long to fix it, after all it isn't the worst thing that has happened. Dad would never know. My feeble efforts were failing to thaw out the pipes. As much as I wanted to keep Dad from knowing about this, I had to call him.

Shortly afterwards David Gidcumb (mom and dad's pastor) showed up. We looked at the well house and determined where the pipes had frozen. He made some calls and said he was going to run and grab a small heater. A few minutes after David left, there was a knock on the door and Sandy Stephens showed up with a heater. We worked for a while and got the water going to the well house but no water to the house. After much deliberation we tried to crawl under the house. Now those of you that know me know that I "ain't as skinny as I once was". The last time that I went under the house I was half my age and half my size. We couldn't get through the crawl space. We pretty much determined that it was not something we could handle. We talked for a few minutes and Sandy went back up to collect his tools.

I stepped back in to call Dad and tell him that the pipes had frozen under the house. I had just told him that when I heard the sound of water gushing out of the faucet. WE HAD WATER.

I hung up and yelled at Sandy that we had water. What had been impossible was happening.

There is no doubt in my mind that God was with us today. We can read in several places in the Bible where God sent men to go to those in trouble and to deliver them. Two of those men came to me today. No thought of self-gain, but rather seeing their brother in trouble and wanting to help. Living that great commandment to love one another. Throughout the past several months there have been many who have stepped in to help in so many ways that I don't know about, whether it was stopping by to see Mom and Dad, to bringing firewood, or sitting with Mom while Dad was on the road.

I want all of you to know that we appreciate it. You have shown that in this dreary world there are still those who want to do what is right, to show love to their brothers and sisters.

I can't complain about today when in every situation, God showed he was in control and that everything would be ok, from Dr. Voight coming in and telling us that the surgery went well and that Mom would be okay to the wonderful sound of water flowing in the sink.

Thanks to all and I pray that God is with you and looks over you as He has for my family.

Wes Weber

January 8th Posted by Wesley

I talked with Mom this morning. She is doing well and seemed upbeat. The Doctor was in to see her this morning and they both felt she should stay there for another night to be on the safe side. She is at PCRMC Room 307 for those who were asking about dropping by or calling. By Wes Weber

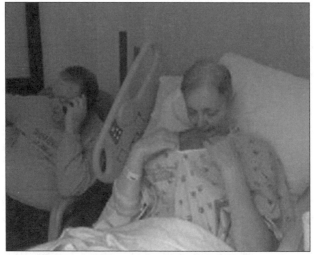

Wonder what they did down there??

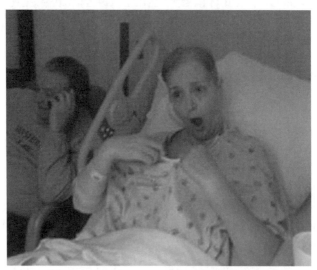

**Oh my goodness... they did what!!!!!
(Blame it on the medication!!!)**

Chop! Chop! The Chopping Block!

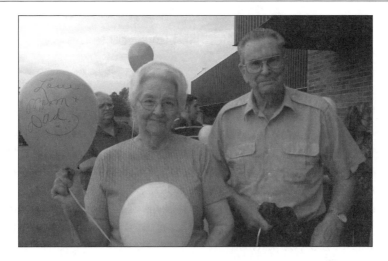

My parents at my balloon lift off! Please send up special prayers for them. They lost one daughter to ovarian cancer. This makes my breast cancer double hard on them. Please pray for them!!

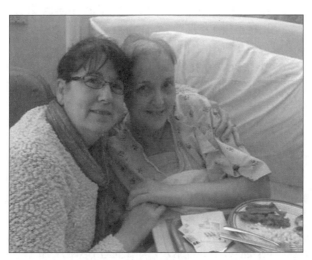

Goodness!
I look at pictures like this and now understand why so many felt bad for me. Did I really look this bad! Should have had my bad hair day hat on!!
My sister Jill and me!

The Pink Duck

> A note from my baby sister Jill. I love you to the moon and back!
>
> I have come to believe that having only 2 sisters is like having only 2 eyes. When you lose one, you only have one left, and you want to protect it and take care of it like never before!!! I hate what my sister is going through! I don't like to see her hurt! She is strong, but I will ride this roller coaster with her thru every needle, every test, every tear, and every lost hair! Together we will dance in the rain and hug thru the pain! I am here for you always, my dearest sister! I love you, Karen!!

It's funny the things that pop into your head when you're under stress or on funny meds! I got to wondering if I should take a before and after picture!!! But, I couldn't frame it or put it in a photo album. I couldn't even tuck it in a picture box to run across later. Blame the thought on the meds. It didn't make sense to me either. I'm still on funny meds so please don't hold me accountable for what I write tonight!

In spite of the somber situation here we have done some silly laughing and I'm not sure I even know what's funny! Or what's not funny for that matter! We had to get up at 4 a.m. Tuesday morning to get here on time. Now that was NOT funny! Neither was the drive at -12 degrees on the ice covered roads.

I had a whole party here to pray over me and hug me before going off to surgery. It has touched my heart that so many would get up so early and drive on ice covered roads in freezing temperatures to be here for Joe and me!

I'm sure the chopping block was as scary as it sounds but I don't remember any of it. I was in good hands and know there were angels in the room and I certainly was covered in prayer. I've done really well even though as is to be expected, I am SORE! The drain bulbs are certainly a new experience as is my new swollen shape. My room has been full of wonderful friends and family visitors and beautiful flowers. The staff here at the hospital have been wonderful! I have been so blessed. How can one person have so many blessings poured out on them??? I am so thankful for your many prayers and post of encouragement. When I don't have weird thoughts running through my mind, I'm praying for you too!! Hoping to go home tomorrow.

Apparently I did talk quite a bit after surgery. In the recovery room, I told the nurses I thought they should mop the floor. Later I asked them if they'd got the floor mopped!

Silly me!

January 9th, 2014

I am totally blank tonight, but I do want to let you know I am HOME and doing great!! I ended up staying another day at the hospital because neither my DR nor I felt comfortable with my going home. I am about as sore as a person can get. There was a lot to learn before coming home. I must say I'm glad they put you on medication because I'm not sure a person could deal with it all otherwise. That's big coming from someone who doesn't take anything for pain other than a coke and dark chocolate.

I was right down pathetic when they unwrapped my bandages but my dear sweet husband who has been constantly by my side told me to not worry about it that, "I've got this honey!" Whatever that means, it sure made me feel better. I guess I was expecting to see healed well defined scars. That's not what I saw. We won't even go there. What I do know; barring any bad reports coming back from the lab... I am down to a 1% chance of getting breast cancer again. That my friends is worth jumping up out of your seats and doing the Happy Dance.

You would not believe the party we are planning for this spring/summer when this is all over. You will be invited!!! I want to give a special shout out to DR VOIGHT and all of the nurses, aides, and staff at the hospital who did their very best to help and encourage us. Especially those who raced us up and down the hall as we made our little walks!!! Surviving and thriving!

Please pray for our oldest son Timothy Weber. He's in ICU on a ventilator with double pneumonia in North Dakota!!! This mama is very concerned as he's really been sick the past few days and they just admitted him to the hospital. We are trying to get more information now. Pray for his family also as some of them have been sick too.

January 10th, 2014

Timothy's nurse said they are going to do test tomorrow, an ultrasound on his heart and a camera in his lungs. With the camera they will use water to break up the congestion. His nurse said his lungs are saturated. The camera will help them know more about what is going on. Thank you for praying!!!!

January 11th, 2014

I've really been a little too stressed to be on here, what with being concerned about our son Timothy and adjusting here at the house with me. Thank you for praying for both of us. Timothy is still in ICU and on the ventilator. He will remain on it for a few more days. I talked with his nurse today and she said he is in good spirits. He can't talk because of the ventilator but his wife called and put the phone on speaker so I could talk to him. I told him I guess he'd learned not to talk back and of course he smiled over that! They have to keep him somewhat sedated so he doesn't cough and pull the tubes out of him.

As for me... I'm doing really well. I don't look my best but I smell good! I was excited to get a shower today! I've had a bit of pain today and had to take more medication for it. I am so blessed to have a sister-in-law helping me and encouraging me on. She has been a real trooper as has Joe. My home health nurse (Melinda Rathburn) came yesterday and helped me through some more of my grieving process and taught us how to change the bandages etc.

Chop! Chop! The Chopping Block!

I am so thankful for each of you who have encouraged me and prayed for me. You'll never know how much it really means to me!!! I love you each and pray for you too. Some of you (dare I say all of you) are going through your own special rough spots. We are remembering you in your time of need too. Isn't is awesome that we have a Father that sees all!!

Three of my greatest blessings in life are my sons! Our oldest son is Timothy Joseph. Some people call him Tim but if you ask him, he'll tell you he prefers to be called Timothy. That's what we call him too. After all he was named after Timothy in the bible and also after his dad (Joe) He was premature at birth. Weighing in at 4 1/2 pounds. Now he's about 6'2" or more. He's a "happy go lucky" personality. He has four beautiful children. Three girls and our only grandson. They just live way too far from us!! (North Dakota) TJ works with the oil fields. Timothy can give some of the best ever bear hugs!

We brought our second blessing home on Timothy's 2nd birthday! I'm not sure Timothy was too pleased with a baby brother for a birthday present but we decided to keep him anyway. Wesley Mark... he took his dad's middle name and we gave him Wesley just because we loved the name. He however prefers to be called "Wes". Wes has always been one who loved life. If there is action... that's where you'll find Wes. He's been in about every line of law enforcement out there from deputy to Kansas Hwy Patrol to Undersheriff. Right now he attends Washburn Law School. I need to give a shout out for him getting all B's this semester, as did our youngest son James Kelly (named after my two grandfathers) but better known as Jake.

Jake is our only child who wasn't pre-mature. He's a big 6'4" at least and attends Washburn Law School too. Congratulations on your all B's too. Jake is the daddy to Thing One and Thing Two. We are blessed that they live close to us. I love our mother/son days! Jake and I share a birthday month and love to shop together and celebrate our month together. Yep, we take the whole month!!! We are so blessed to have these three big hearted sons. They give the best bear hugs ever!!! When they are all three at our house you'll hear a lot of laughter and giggling.... "Can you top this?'....and "take that!!!" How I love my boys!!

January 12th, 2014

Not the best day (still struggling with pain) but we were still blessed. Thank you Tony & Sarah Parks for the wonderful Sunday Dinner. We so appreciated it. Please keep our son Timothy in your prayers. He's still in ICU. They had to keep him sedated today to keep him from being so restless and irritated with the tubes from the ventilator. It sounds like he's not coming off of it as soon as they had hoped. I so wish we were able to be there with him. Thank you for your prayers. Praying you are all well and keeping away from the flu etc. out there!! RUN!!!

January 13th, 2014

I woke up in a weepy state this morning. I don't know why that happens but it does sometimes. It's not my nature to be so weepy. My first thoughts were self-pity. It seems when you are in pain it becomes "all about me" real quick!!

I just felt like I'd been robbed of so much. Robbed of my health, robbed of my good blood cells, robbed of my looks, robbed of my hair, robbed of my body parts, robbed of healthy looking skin... robbed of my peace of mind. I felt robbed of my time with Thing One and Thing Two... robbed of getting to travel with Joe...robbed of getting to do my own grocery shopping. Robbed of my energy... I was really in a state of mind! I just gave you the "short list".

Our preacher's wife (Cathy Gidcumb) called me and even though I was fine when she called, just the fact that she called to see how I was and if I had a prayer request for the staff meeting...made me weepy. Of course then I felt silly for being such a "weep"!! They must have prayed hard for me because the next thing I knew; my day was feeling better.

I began to receive one blessing after another. I got to have my first shower since hitting the chopping block. Oh! What a blessing! I've lost count of the times Joe has come up behind my chair and bent down and put a kiss on top of my bald head!!! With these tubes coming out of me we can't even hug!!!

Joe and Theresa and I sat down and was talking today and ended up laughing and laughing. What a blessing to have laughter in our house!!! I got a beautiful basket of flowers from my brother-in-law who had been married to the sister we'd lost to ovarian cancer. What a sweet surprise. I also received a wonderful unexpected phone call from Timothy's best friend calling to check on me! I so enjoyed our visit!!!

My sister and her husband came and brought Pizza Inn pizza for lunch today! I was even able to play a song on the piano! I haven't played the piano since Sept! I found myself singing today! Psalm 40 v 3 "He put a new song in my mouth, a hymn of praise to our God." Thank you everyone for your prayers for Timothy and me.

Timothy is still on the ventilator. He was not able to do ok on his own today when they tried to take him off of it. They had to sedate him again to keep him from being agitated and pulling the tubes out. How I wish they were closer so some of us (family) could go see him and encourage him. He is really having it rough. This really stresses me!!!

Job 42 v 10 "after Job had prayed for his friends, the Lord made him prosperous again and gave him twice as much as he had before." How can we ever repay you each for praying for us??? It's not in our power but we pray the Lord will bless each of you abundantly!!! I know the prayers of others changed my day as when I woke, I really didn't feel like praying!!! I was too self-absorbed. I thank God for those who intercede when I struggle!!!! I truly am humbled by your traveling with me on this journey! Even when I have grown bone weary, you have not!! I thank you from the bottom of my heart!

January 14th, 2014

Update on Timothy... Timothy is still under the weather. Michelle called today and said he will still have to be on the ventilator for several days. His lungs are swollen and irritated and he can only breathe on his own 50% of the time. He has been on the ventilator five days now. If he has to be on it another five days they will have to look at putting in a tracheal tube. They are trying to stretch his lungs which are still inflamed and infected. He has made a little headway but it's been very slow. As the nurse told me... he was very ill when he arrived at the hospital. He has been very agitated and frustrated at the tubes down his throat and has tried to pull them out so they have to keep him sedated. Please pray for a quick full recovery. If you have a prayer team please add him. Thank you very much and may you be blessed abundantly!!! Happy 5th birthday to their 3rd child Abby Dabby Doo! We love you baby doll!

Blood work back on Timothy. He also has Influenza A on top of the double pneumonia.

January 15th, 2014

Good news on Timothy! They were able to pull the tube today and he's doing well. I just talked with his nurse and she said they'd had him sitting up today and he was able to eat a little bit. She said they would probably be moving him to a different floor and out of ICU in the near future. She felt like he'd made a turn for the better. When he wakes up, I can call his cell phone and talk to him! YIPPEE!!!! Thank you all for putting him on your prayer list! Prayer is a mighty source of power and we believe whole heartedly in it.

For myself... I too have had a good day. Not as much pain as yesterday. I am going to go in there and try to make a batch of no bake cookies that someone put on the internet and made me hungry for. Ok... so Theresa is probably going to make them and I'm going to watch. Maybe she'll let me lick the spoon! I'm feeling blessed to have such a prayer team support and a Father in heaven who listens to our pleadings and answers. So many of you have cried tears with us and we have cried with you on your sorrows too. So many of you are facing mountains also!!! We are so thankful for each of you. You are still in our prayers.

I talked briefly to Timothy tonight. It was hard for him to talk and he wasn't feeling too good. But he's heading in the right direction!!

January 16th, 2014

We are excited to hear Timothy was moved out of ICU today. He's still on oxygen but we haven't heard more yet. For myself, I do not want a repeat of my experience today! I had my first visit with the surgeons since leaving the hospital. I had my drains removed; which I was tremendously excited to have removed. Oh my word, that is not something I ever want to go thru again. No way! No way! No way!!!! I thought I was going to come unglued. Joe said it looked like they were starting up a lawn mower when they told me to cough and then pulled the drains out. I was concerned because I thought all along that they were in me about 2 inches. I would really have croaked if I'd known they were about 36 inches or more!!! Mercy... mercy!!!! I am glad that is over with!!! Oh my!!!!!

I did not get the most exciting news on my labs. The cancer apparently reached further then they expected and there was more cancer in the lymph nodes. I'll learn more at my DR appointment tomorrow morning. I was told today that because of the lab results that they would need to take a more aggressive approach to my treatment. I'm not for sure what all that is going to entail. Tonight I really do feel good. We're going to take this one day at a time. Thanks for walking with me on this journey!!

January 18th, 2014

Do you want the good news or the bad news first? The good news is.... Timothy got to go home today. We haven't heard anything since the text saying he was being dismissed. We did get to talk to him last night and he sounded a lot better and his good humor was back in tact, though he won't be able to return to work for a couple of weeks.

As for me.... I would have thrown a fit except we had a house full of company and I'm too much of a lady to throw a big fit in public. I did feel like it though. I truly had a battle with the mind. Those of you who know me; know that I do not say bad words. I had to keep telling my mind to not go there!!! I was so angry, so devastated, so mad, so let down, so hurt!!!!

How do you handle your body turning on yourself! It wasn't anybody's fault. Just my own body silently betraying me. It made me angry! It's one thing for someone else to betray you... but when you betray yourself, that's another story!

I was called into the DR office because my cancer DR did not want to give me bad news on the phone. They received my lab reports in from my surgery. Sixteen out of sixteen lymph nodes had cancer in them. In my first surgery only one out of three nodes were affected. This totally took the surgeon and cancer team by surprise. They said it was unexpected because I'm so healthy and that they had not seen this before.

This means that first off I will have to chase down Butterscotch (the neighbor's cat) and have another PET scan. I'm not sure how he's going to feel about that, as he wasn't too happy about the last one! After that I will have aggressive and well monitored 12 weeks straight of chemo and then.... (What I didn't want) radiation. We aren't sure how much or how long. But treatment will be longer than we expected. Needless to say, I'm very disappointed.

Keep walking along beside me and we'll still dance in the rain. It won't be in April as previously planned, but maybe a summer rain. In any case, I'll keep praying for you too!!

January 19th, 2014

This morning the first thing Joe said to me was, "Do you feel like church this morning?" I promptly said "yes", but I didn't get ready because I didn't want to go. I felt too bald and too scarred. I felt like everything showed. I decided I'd just stay home until my hair grew back out and my skin improved. So... I didn't get ready.

Joe came in and sat down in his chair. "Aren't you going to church?" I asked him. He answered that he would just stay home with me instead. I realized my pride was keeping us both from going, so I jumped up and said I would go with him. We only had about 20 minutes to get ready!

I grabbed my new wig (which I'm sure I'll never get used to) instead of a scarf. I chose the wig because I didn't have a scarf to match my outfit. In my world things have to match. We headed out the door. We were about five minutes late and as we walked in the door, my attitude still had not changed. I felt bald with a cat sitting on my head. I felt flat! I did not want to be there.

I wasn't two feet inside the door when I began receiving hugs from some of my favorite people. It just made me weepy and I still wanted to just go back home even though I really appreciated the hugs. (You know who you are and you know I love you!!!!) I just hate being weepy.

We went on into the sanctuary and our worship leader was saying "We are thankful we aren't where we were!" I wasn't sure about that! I liked where I was more than where I am.

A year ago I was active, alive, busy, and extremely happy! I was leading bible studies for ladies. I had hair and my whole body was intact. I can honestly say I'm not sure I'm glad I'm where I am now compared to where I was. Maybe in a year, I can say I'm thankful I'm not where I was!

I know I was probably missing the whole point. Maybe I was missing it on purpose. Our pastor said something that really touched my heart. He said "The expression on our face, tells a lot about our journey!" Lord, help me with this!!! I have joy for the Lord and I want it to shine, but it wasn't shining too much until we sat under the sound of His word this morning.

I'm so thankful Joe didn't walk out the door without me this morning. In the parking lot Joe asked me where I'd like to eat.

I answered "Chili's". That's an hour and a half from home!! So we headed out. We picked up my sister and her husband and they went with us! Jill and I shopped at one store because I couldn't handle more and then we headed home. It was a great, great day! That's what listening to the word of God can do for you.

January 21st. 2014

Life can be funny sometimes! Sunday my sister and I went to Dress Barn to buy some camisoles. I no longer have a reason to wear a bra! That's odd! I'll have to wear camisoles instead.

    I was trying on a top in the dressing room. I still can't raise my left arm much, so it's hard to get in and out of tops. I also had my wig on. The ladies there led us to the dressing room with our names on our doors.

    I was having a hard time trying the top on so I took my wig off, laid it aside and finally was able to get the top on. I was going to get my sister's opinion of how it looked. I opened the door to show her. One of the ladies that was waiting on us went to ask me how I was doing and completely went blank as she stood there and stared at me. She tried to recover quickly but I was already laughing. The lady who she thought went in the dressing room wasn't who she saw standing there. I got a kick out of it. I can see where I can have some fun with this wig thing!

    I'm so excited about my new idea!! We have a wall in our home that we are going to have the names of everyone who has been praying for us put on that wall!!! You might call it our own prayer wall!!! But YOUR name is going to be on it!!! We are so thankful for each of you who have been cheering me on and praying for us. Your encouragement has been so helpful to us. You have lifted us day after day. Your post humble me!!! We haven't figured out exactly how we are going to do it but we have chosen what wall we are going to do it on. If any of you have any cool ideas; let me hear them!!! There will literally be hundreds of names on the wall. I've been feeling great the past three days. I've been able to get out and even got to drive my car! Waaa Hooo! We got to be with Thing One and Thing Two. I kicked up my heels today and then had to come in and take a pain pill. It was probably too much cold air for my surgery but I sure enjoyed my Joe and Karen day!!!

January 23rd, 2014

I need to get some things done around here but I'm slower than the seven year itch and six years behind on scratching! Every time I try getting something done, well let's just say... I'm not making much headway! I'm getting a little impatient with myself! I wish I still looked like the girl in my profile picture! Taken less than a year ago!!!

Bored???? Nope, I'm just sitting here waiting for the bread machine to go off so I can slap a stick of butter on the end piece and eat it before I go to bed! I've been as moody today as a Missouri thermometer! Am I the only one? One minute I'm up; the next I'm down. That's not normally me. Who is this woman in my chair!!!

January 29th, 2014

It's been a very hectic week and I haven't had a chance to be on here much. I did want to let you all know that I will be having a CAT scan on Friday a.m. I was supposed to have a PET scan so they could compare apples to apples from my last PET scan. However, the insurance company knows best and won't pay for a PET scan and instead wants me to do the CAT scan. So I'm out here chasing the neighbor's cat again. Here kitty kitty!

Joe had to pick up some kind of kit at the hospital today so I can start drinking three huge drinks of "stuff". It doesn't look like something I would choose from the menu. The difference between the PET scan and the CAT scan is the CAT scan stretches over the whole body area.

I'm asking you to please pray that I won't have a bad reaction to/from the test, and that the cancer has not moved to any other area. Pray they DID get it all with the surgery and that I'm well on my way to recovery.

On the flip side, I have been doing fabulous all week!!! It's been a super good week and has really given me hope and encouragement. I have two DR appointments after the CAT scan FRIDAY. One with my cancer DR and one with my surgeon. I just want FABULOUS reports!!! You just keep praying for me and I'll keep praying for you and your family!!! We'll give God the Praise!! Love you bunches

January 30th, 2014

Ok, this might be a little embarrassing for me but it's been a part of my journey and goes in my journal so I'm sharing. You have to promise me though, that you won't cry. I already did that, enough for all of us. Look at it with humor and just chuckle along with me. (I can do that now) Besides that, it was last week. It happened exactly a week ago so it's water (muddy) under the bridge. It was my first time that Joe had to be away. I was doing just fine. I was still quite sore but fine, none the less.

You know when you are on a roller coaster you don't always know where the ups and downs and curves are. That's supposed to be part of the fun although you'll never find me getting on a roller coaster on purpose!!! I don't like them and I didn't choose this one! Joe had to teach in Kansas this week and had a three day trip planned. I was feeling good enough (I thought) that I would go along with him. After all I haven't been out much since September. With chemo starting up again next week; it seemed the ideal time to take a trip with Joe before I started back on bull riding.

I had it all planned out. He was going to St. Joe to the home office. I just love all of the people he works with so I was very excited to get to go to the home office with him. Tuesday he had to educate at a new jail in Kansas which just happens to be located in a town about 40 miles from where my best friend of thirty nine years lives.

Sherry was going to come and pick me up. We were going to eat at our favorite place in town and talk each other's ear off!!! On the way from Kansas, Joe and I was going to stop and have supper with our two sons (Wes and Jake) and spend the evening with them. An exciting time for sure!! I tell you all of this so you will see how important this trip was to me.

Thursday of last week I found out the weather was going to be way too cold for me to venture out with my already irritated scars. I was disappointed to say the least but I could deal with it until I got on the computer and found out my journal (YES. MY JOURNAL that I share with you) had completely disappeared except for two post (from my computer)!!!

I lost it!!! I started crying...and crying... and crying. I was so upset! I went to the bathroom to wash off my face. Those of you who know me know that I can have a party any place. If there's only two of us; well it can still be a party!

I was washing my hands and face and happened to look up and low and behold, right there in the mirror was somebody to have a party with. (A pity party that is) I noticed the lady in the mirror had tears on her (only eight) eye-lashes left. She looked so sad and pitiful that I felt sorry for her and started to really cry.

Have you ever seen someone in the mirror cry??? I don't know who she was but my crying must have really bothered her and she really started crying. Which made me cry and so we went in one vicious cycle. Me crying... her crying... me crying... her crying...

I cried because of her hair, her chopped body, her poor little eight eyelashes, and dry skin. I cried because my journal was gone and because it was too cold for me to go on the trip. I cried because I couldn't go to the home office and missed out on Olive Gardens in St. Joe. I cried because I was going to miss eating at Heavy's BBQ out in Kansas. I cried because I wasn't going to get to eat at Carlos O Kelly's in Salina with Sherry! I wasn't going to get to eat with Wes and Jake and Joe and laugh until we were sore!

I cried because the lady in the mirror cried and she cried because I looked so bad crying with her. I cried because she looked so bad crying with me! In all of this excitement I accidently broke a nail! I've never in my life cried over a broken nail, but I did then. The lady in the mirror cried over it too. It was a big deal last week, but it's not this week.

This week, I got to feel those fun belly dips on the roller coaster. Monday my friend (Amy Green) came over and helped me with house cleaning that I couldn't do. It was awesome to see the floors shine and the sweeper run. It was wonderful to see the dust disappear from the furniture! We chatted and laughed all day long!! Tuesday my parents came and brought cabbage rolls and we got to spend the day together. Another friend brought me Tacos for supper and spent the evening. Wednesday, my cousin came (who also had had surgery) and we got to go to Pizza Inn and spend the afternoon together. We filled up on Pizza and Cinnamon Stromboli and then came home and ate popcorn and Hershey bars!!

Today is a peaceful day where I get to rest and catch up from all of this week's excitement! We're having stuffed peppers prepared by Ahleesha Elwood, another friend (for our supper) YUM!! At nine o'clock tonight I start drinking "the stuff" and preparing for another dip on the roller coaster. (The dreaded PET scan) The neighbor's cat hasn't been around all day!! Wonder why!!!

Drink one down!!! UGH...It took me one hour and 15 minutes. That can't happen tomorrow!! I have to drink one at 7 a.m. and one at 8 a.m. At least it doesn't taste as bad as I expected!!

January 31st, 2014

Well it's been a day, it has!!! I drank my TWO bottles of "the stuff". We headed to the hospital to take the CAT scan. I couldn't find the neighbor's cat, so I didn't have anyone to stand in for me and had to face the dip on the roller coaster myself.

It wasn't as bad as I feared and I didn't react to the dye used. They even let Joe in to hold my hand!!! You would NOT believe the big chicken I am when I face anything like this. I will buy a new piece of clothing rather than sew a button on, because I am so afraid of needles!!! Not really, but you do get the picture, don't you!!!

After the CAT scan we headed to get me a bottle of water because I was so dry from not being able to drink anything from 9 p.m. the night before. But, I'm dragging my story out. I have something exciting to tell you!!!

We went on to the see DR Nevils. Oh happy, happy, happy day!!! She had the results from my CAT scan and said there was NO cancer found in the rest of my body!!! Talk about excited!!!! I am! I am! I am!! I start chemo Tuesday for 12 weeks straight and then radiation for 4 - 7 weeks after that. This is to prevent the cancer from returning. Afterwards I will be on a pill for five years to control the estrogen. Estrogen is what drives the cancer.

After the first DR appointment, we went over to the Lord's Library and to my surprise there was a surprise party awaiting me. Ladies from my bible study group had gathered to surprise me. My friend Loretta Phelps had made me a beautiful quilt. They had a dinner prepared and several surprises. What a wonderful surprise and a wonderful time!

After the party I had an appointment with my surgeon. Do you know what he told me? He told me that I'm way ahead of the game!! He said that even though my CAT scan said that I was "unremarkable" (which is what we want it to say) that I was remarkable anyway! Sweet huh! He said I am healing from surgery faster that most do. I could move in more directions and reach higher than most people at my stage of recovery. I guess all those days of laying on the floor pounding my fist and stomping my feet has paid off!!! They want me to stay on the Melaleuca vitamins and to keep doing what I'm doing, because it's working!!!

We got to have Thing One and Thing Two here with us for supper. Although tonight I am exhausted from such a wonderful day, I am praising God for praying friends and family!!! Thank you for your prayers!!! We reached the throne!!

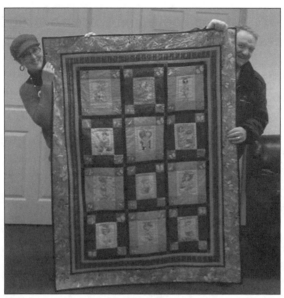

**Beautiful Cancer Quilt made for me by Loretta Phelps
Joe and Karen
At my surprise party!**

Chapter 6

Back On the Bull
(It's anything but normal)

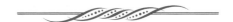

February 1st, 2014

I am thinking of Joe's cousin today and his family in the loss of his sweet wife. Pam battled breast cancer which spread to other areas. She fought a long hard battle and we will all miss her. RIP, wife, mother, daughter, sister, granddaughter, cousin, aunt, niece, friend and neighbor. Your life touched so many lives.

WOW! I'm working on rebuilding my journal. It's a good thing I gave my parents a copy since they aren't on face book. However, it only goes up to my surgery day. (To bad I didn't remember that on the day I had my "come apart"!) I could have saved the lady in the mirror and myself a lot of anguish!

I'm also working on getting everyone's name in the book so I can start on my prayer wall. Oh my goodness, now that's going to be a big job and I can't wait to get 'er done! I love seeing your names over and over! The prayer wall just keeps growing and growing! Who says people no longer pray!!!!! You all are such a powerful group here! Might I suggest we pray for our country also!! Maybe we just better make it the WORLD! After all we have several of you from other countries on here too!!! I am amazed at your faithfulness!!! I appreciate your prayers! I'm still loving to pray for you!!!

February 3rd, 2014

I'm gearing up to get back on the bull tomorrow. UGH! I am not looking forward to it! It will be a different chemo, but the same fantastic group of nurses and DR. I've had such a wonderful week this week. I was able to do several fun things even if my energy doesn't last all day yet.

Yesterday my sister and I went to K Mart to check on hats for me. If you have never gone hat shopping, let me tell you, don't ever just walk in and pull a hat off the rack and expect it to fit! They come in all sizes. One size does not fit all!!! We took about six or seven different hats back to the dressing room to try on. Only one really fit. (Some might say... I only have one head, so one (hat) ought to be enough) I on the other hand like my hats to match my outfits. We went back to check out more hats.

The guys were sitting in the car eating Wendy's frosties and guarding the two frosties we had bought to drop off for mom and dad. About the time Jill and I got back to the hats again, we both got a text from the guys saying... "Frosties are melting!"

I had more hats in my hands to try on and it was halfway across the store to the dressing room. So I just grabbed my wig off and we started running around looking for mirrors. There was none in sight. Finally it was just prudent to just go back to the dressing room. We were running across the store, hats in hands. I had my wig in my other hand, bald head just a shining!!! We were laughing ourselves silly. I'm surprised the bells and whistles didn't go off when we left the store.

It was so cold outside that when we got back to the car, the boys had set the ice cream outside to keep it from melting!!

Today Thing One and Thing Two were here. We were brushing our teeth and putting our make up on and Thing One said, "OH! You have to put your hair on too!" I replied, "Awww... do I have to wear it today? It's hot! Can I just not wear anything today?!" She looked at me with a sparkle in her eyes and said: "I love you bald head!" Of course, Thing Two had to imitate her! Yep! I was rolling on the floor laughing!

I plan on pounding that bull tomorrow. Please help me out by keeping me in your prayers and I'll keep praying for you!

It was a wonderful afternoon. Thing One, Thing Two and myself! We were having a "tea party" at the pretend McDonalds in the girls' room. We had PJ "samages", grapes and lemon cobweb cake. We had hardly sat down when, "ring ring"... the girl's toy phone rang and Thing One jumped up to answer it! "Hello...yes... yes we can... WOW! Uh huh...uh huh... yes, I'll tell them! Ok!"

I asked her, "Was that someone important?" She answered "No, not really, it was just Penny!" (Her imaginary friend) She continued, "After our tea party we're going on a Pool Run!"

Me: "What's a pool run?"

Thing One "It's when you have a big thing and you slide down in the swimming pool! We're going to all put on our swim suits and go to the beach!"

I said: "Are you sure about that? It's pretty cold outside!" (Remember it is February!)

She stepped out of the bed room into the hallway and raised her arms up in the air! She said: "Ohhhhh it's beautiful out here!!! It's nice and warm!!!"

We ate our lunch and got the "blue" blankets out and laid them out on our almost white carpet in the living room. The girls put fake snowballs on the blankets to make it look like bubbles.

We were all to be mermaids!!! That means we had to keep our legs and feet together at all times!!! Thing One said her name was "Elsa" and that I could be "Rapunzel'. I looked at Thing Two and asked: "what is your name?' She looked at me as though I'd lost a marble or two and in surprise said "My name is Thing Two!" Ok!! How could I not know that!!

We continued to play. We pretended to swim and wiggled around and tossed imaginary bubbles! All of a sudden right in the middle of playing Thing One went "Whoo! Whooo"! She asked me if I knew what THAT was.

I said "No. What was it?"

She said "It was an owl! It's our bedtime!" So we closed our eyes and got comfortable!

I was really getting into enjoying myself when she crowed like a rooster!!! I opened one eye and would have been content with a longer than a one minute nap, but no, we had to jump up and get right back at playing mermaids tossing imaginary bubbles! That my friend is how you play with kids!!! I know you understand why these girls are my sunshine!!!!

February 4th, 2014

Waiting to be called in for chemo. Thank you Joe for always being here to hold my hand!!!! You give me strength and courage every time!

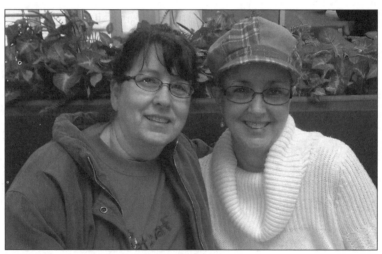

Jill and Karen

My faithful sister shows up at every chemo treatment with a new home made card for me, cheering me on. She also gave up her Mondays off so she could be there to support me on Tuesdays when Joe can't be there. What kind of sister gives up her Mondays for her sister? ONLY the BEST! I love you to the moon and back Jill-Re!!!!

February 6th, 2014

Have you ever been in a room where chemo is given? It's a little different. It's always a full house for sure! People sitting around visiting, eating, knitting, reading books, sleeping! You see it all. But they all have one thing in common. Their bodies have attacked them in one form or another.

Each time I arrive at the chemo room, I immediately look around the room to see if the same familiar faces are there? Who is new, who is scared, who unsure, who is resigned? Who looks better this week?

This week there was a missing man. He's been there every time that I've been there and has often been in the chair across from me. Close to my age, I suspect. Tall and slender. Always quiet and to himself. They buried him last week. For some reason it hit me like a ton of bricks! I learned that he had stage 4 lung cancer. That is was too late by the time they found it. I wondered why he took chemo. But I know it's the HOPE. It's the hope of spending more time with our families. The hope of getting better!!! The hope of not giving up! The thought that I'm not just doing this for me, but I'm doing this for you my family and friends too! My heart goes out to his family! To his wife!

My eyes continue around the room. There's new faces here. Some have lost their hair already. Other's will soon. I know how they feel! However, this room isn't a dreary room. It's full of hope and the nurses and doctors are always so cheerful! They are truly gifted and full of love for their patients. I'm impressed with the encouragement they give each person there.

If you ever get a chance to go sit with someone getting chemo, I suggest you go! You will be blessed!! A new world will open up to you! Your eyes will be opened to prayer needs for sure! But you'll also be encouraged! If you see someone who doesn't have anyone sitting beside them, sit down beside them and hear their story! Everyone in there has a different one and they are all interesting! They are all precious! I pray for you that you will never have to know chemo for yourself! That you will be blessed with good health! But if you do get sent down this path, it doesn't mean the blessings stop! They're just from a different perspective. God is always good!

February 7th, 2014

OH my!!! I'm not happy about this pain! I'm hoping it's not just the new chemo. I wonder if the cold weather is compounding it.

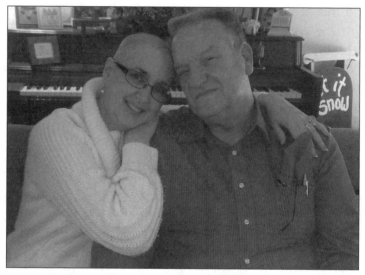

My Sweetheart and Me!!

February 10th, 2014

Last week was kind of rough after riding the bull. I get back on him tomorrow and of course I dread that! It really started hitting me about Thursday evening and I was almost in tears by Friday. This time instead of being so tired it hit my bones with pain. However Saturday it eased up and I was able to really enjoy a visit from my two special nieces (April & Adora and little Zander).

The girls are my sister's (who we lost to ovarian cancer 11 years ago) children. It was a bitter sweet visit because they remind me of Lynn and I remind them of their mother. So we'd laugh a while and then cry a while, laugh some more and cry some more!

Thing One and Thing Two came and spent Sunday night and all day today with us!!! Oh we love those girls! I'm not sure how much Thing One thinks I've lost since being diagnosed. We were talking about how things will be different this summer when I start growing hair again and we can play outside in the sand box. She said to me, "Nana if you still have your brain and can remember we can build a sandcastle and put diamonds and seashells on it!!!" Say WHAT?? IF, I still have my brain? I wonder where she got that!

Thing Two ran a fever today and wasn't feeling too good, but about every 10 minutes she would say to me, "I still love you Nana!"

Thing One was in Joe's office looking around and she said to him, "Were you a cop before you did the job you do now?" He answered "yes" he was. She said, "Wow! That's pretty impressive!! You're pretty awesome!"

Life is good! God is good all the time!!! We dropped by Common Grounds for supper tonight! Thank you to whoever slipped and paid for our supper! We were surprised when we went up to pay, but thankful!!!! May blessings rain down upon you and your family!! Thanks for praying for us! We are praying for you too!!!! I'm collecting names for my prayer wall! It's going to be awesome!!!

February 12th, 2014

Joe and I were so blessed with all of the comments and private chats we received after posting our picture of my bald self. You my friends are amazing!!! Your encouragement to us and how you are also encouraging one another in this journey is blessing so many!!! Each and every post is wonderfully rolled around in our hearts, hugged and treasured.

If you look up all of the references to a bald head in the bible you might get discouraged! It can however be an interesting read! I prefer to look at the cup as overflowing! In my new bible I was looking in the dictionary - concordance pages for the word bald. I could not even find the word but the word beauty stood out instead on the page where bald should have been. I took it as an omen to follow that line of thinking instead!

I had to go back to some of my older bibles with more extended concordance to even find the word bald or baldness. I'll leave it to you to trail that path if you'd like some interesting reads. The "bald head" came up again this week in several different situations.

Thing One and Thing Two were here and of course it's going to come up with them around. Thing One has finally come to terms with my not having hair. She loves to tease me and say "I love you bald head". Now I might take offence from someone else, but as you know, Thing One, in my sight does not have any faults!!!

The other night she wanted me to sleep beside her. I've started growing "fuzz" on my head and she was lying there rubbing my head. She was so excited to finally get to spend the night again that she was a chatter box and couldn't go to sleep. She started taking a comfort in rubbing my hair (yes I said hair, even if it's only about 1/16th of an inch.) She would rub my head and talk. I'd say "We really need to go to sleep." She would say "Yes, we do! Just one more thing", and then she would hop up again and kiss me on the top of the head!

It's a funny thing about people touching the top of your head! I think a lot of you men without hair might agree with me here. I've seen it happen before and seen several be embarrassed about the situation a person puts them in when someone says "I just want to touch your head!" Say what???? They will duck a bit but still feel caught and still suffer through the head rubbing. I know how you feel. It's like "I'm not a puppy, please keep your hands off my head and don't pat me!!" Space please!! There are people that I will let touch my head.

My mother kissed me on the top of the head Sunday. I felt loved and a little bit like a kid again! Joe has kissed the top of my head many times. He likes to slip around behind my chair and plant a kiss right on top! Yep, I'm feeling the love and he gets points! My sister has also walked behind my chair and planted a kiss. I feel her pain and love as I know how she feels about what I'm going through. After all we both lost our big sister to this crazy cancer monster. You can kiss me there Jill. Even my sister-in-law Theresa planted a kiss on top my head!

My sons have kissed me on the top of my bald head. They are so sweet and I feel sooooo supported and loved each time they kiss me and give me their big ole bear hugs. Yep boys, keep 'em coming! You each mean the world to me!

Thing One and Thing Two will almost make a contest out of who can give me the most kisses on top or the last kiss!!! It makes me happy to get those precious kisses because I know they are accepting the changes in me. I'm just praying this cancer monster will not cause them to grow up and be afraid!! They can say "I love you bald head" to me all they want!!!

We were in the car with the girls waiting for their mama the other night when Thing Two took my wig off and began to rub my head and plant kisses. (I only wear a wig when the girls are around because I don't want this cancer monster to scare them) Other than that, I hate wearing a wig.

Thing Two is such a darling little three year old. When she was done she decided to put the wig back on me. That's a feat for even me and after a try or two and me looking like I had a cat sitting on top; I asked her if she needed a little help. She independently said; "No thank you".

After a few more tries and I think she could pretty much picture the cat sitting up there too, "She humbly said "I do need a little help"! I showed her how you shake it out first and find the tag in the back and wiggle it on your head! Still felt like a cat sitting up there but she was pleased with the results!!!

I believe if you look up beauty instead of bald in the bible you will be encouraged!! The book of Isaiah has some really interesting thoughts! Isaiah 61 is one of my favorite chapters. Isaiah 52 tells us of the lack of beauty in Jesus appearance. Yet we cling to HIM!

I love what Isaiah says in the 38th chapter. Words so long ago but living bread to my soul tonight! You restored me to health and let me live! Surely it was for my benefit that I suffered such anguish. In your love you kept me from the pit of destruction: you have put all my sins behind your back. The living... the living - they praise you, as I am doing today; parents tell their children about your (God's) faithfulness. Oh there's lots more! Just read it!!!

I guess I'll never figure myself out now. For the most part... I'm ok. Then I start looking at pictures. I guess I just need to put the picture boxes away for a while. I was looking at a picture taken a couple of years ago. We were there with another couple. I have hair and a body. Makes me want to cry! Then... I look again and I'm pretty sure I was pinching Joe; so I've got to laugh!

February 17th, 2014

I'm curious. How many times does one have to get on a bull before they are considered to be a professional!!! Of course, I've been kicked off enough that I'm not in the running. It would be nice to win a ribbon sometime though! Make that a crown! I like crowns!!!

Last week's ride was a bit different. My arm and leg muscles wanted to jerk. While walking to the car, I felt a bit drunk. I slept almost entirely through lunch at Gordo's and slept until 6 p.m. that night.

I either dreamed it or my nurse Julie called and said they were going to back down the meds tomorrow. I'm going to have to ask her tomorrow if she called. There are several things about that day that I've been told about and don't remember. After sleeping so much, I was wide awake until 6 in the morning. I finally talked myself into going to sleep because we had to get up at 7 a.m.

My DR let me go (with Joe) on a trip a couple of days to Columbia. We had a lot of fun even though I had to rest quite a bit. I did the day on one hour of sleep though!!! We found a fabulous "organic" store called Lucky's Market there in Columbia!!

Joe and I love grocery stores!!! If you get a chance to go to Lucky's Market; go!!!

I have to say this has been a real good week other than my slow sleepy start! Dinners with friends, time with Thing One and Thing Two and our son James. I even got to work the Welcome Center at church a few minutes!!! As far as writing in my journal; I've been brain dead. Back on the bull tomorrow! I'll never get used to it or like it!! Thanks for your prayers! I'm praying for YOU!!!

February 18th, 2014

Well that bull was chicken today! He even tried to cross the road! Maybe it was because I went in with my boot stompin' boots on. Still he wouldn't let me get on him today. Poor little "scaredy cat"!!! I finally felt like I could go in there with lots of courage. I even had my port plugged in, but no that bull wouldn't let me ride today.

It appears my white blood count was too low. Instead of chemo today I got a SHOT!!! Yep a big long hard one! Again I was a brave girl. I'm sure Joe will attest to it. (High voice... "Huh Joe"... deep low voice..."yup Karen") He only had to put one bandage on the hand I was holding.

Nurse Stephanie explained about these shots to me today. They all are a part of the "Nu or New or some kind of group" Personally I think they should all begin with Wipe. Like "wiped out" because that's what they seem to do to you. I could hardly wait to get back home to my chair!

On the upside we have figured out why Thing One thought I might not still have my brain this summer!! I often say that I have "chemo brain" so I guess she thought it was wiping my brain out! See there's that word again!!!

Today we took her to preschool. She told me "Nana! We need to get through this breast cancer!!" She's so anxious for summer when I'll have hair again. Truth is... I'm already growing hair and eyelashes!!!

My eye lashes are actually longer than my hair but hey, it will all work out in the end. My hair is just fuzz at the moment and I'm not getting too excited about it since this chemo is supposed to take (wipe?) it all out again too.

As it stands Joe won't be able to go with me Thursday to take chemo. Somebody beside me might be surprised when I reach over and grab their hand when Miss Stephanie plugs in my port. I've been thinking how blessed I am to have you all praying for me! I know it has blessed me tremendously to be praying for you!! I'm still working on the names for the prayer wall!!! It's going to be huge! Everyday another name is being added! Every one of you are precious to me! I'm praying God will bless you and yours abundantly!!!

Count down! 10 more to go.... "Ooops"! White blood cells down had to miss chemo!

February 20th, 2014

One of the things chemo can do to you... Is keep you wide awake! It can, I believe make you say things you might not normally share! Kind of like when one has a baby. During labor one might lose their integrity and modestly! But again, my chemo brain talks! I've had about, maybe 3 hours of sleep in the past day and a half! That means I'm losing 14 hours of sleep at this time! UGH! Why can't my eyes close!!

Life has changed at our house so much! It used to be if Joe walked in on me in the bathroom and I wasn't dressed... I would promptly grab my "ammunition" and point them at him and go bang bbbaaaaattttt. No matter how many times it happened, he'd just about fall down laughing. I can't do that now, flat chested as I am, he'd know I was shooting blanks!

Go ahead and laugh, it's funny! We haven't stayed married 38 plus years by not having a lot of laughs!!! I could write a book on that!

I spent the past couple of nights at my folks while Joe was working out of town. Like I said, chemo can keep you wide awake and so it was after three naps during and right after

Back On the Bull (It's anything but normal)

chemo, I was wired for sound and my mother was also wide awake because she'd had a nap too. So.... We ended up talking until after four in the morning!

Although we both gave it our best shot, neither of us was able to completely straighten the other one out. We both laughed and cried through the visit. I was sharing with her some of our experiences that we were going through. Chalk it up to being up late, high on chemo and reaching the too late to pull it back in the conversation point! I shared the experience below with her and she felt like I should share it in my journal. She even tried to help me find the words to delicately say it, but really there isn't any way to say, one night... "I decided to go to bed bare chested!!"

Now you have to understand, Joe has seen my scars! He had to help change bandages on them after surgery. So it's not like anything had been hid. My husband knows every step I have gone through on this rough journey. He has been the trooper! The one with courage!!! The strong one!!! He has not let go of my hand!!! But this night was different. This was the next step on our journey and for some spontaneous reason, I didn't think about doing it before the moment.

I took the next step. I watched his face for his reaction, he watched mine and reached his arms out for me. Now you might tell me as many have said before, these are your battle scars. Be proud of them! Well let me just insert here; though DR Voight is the best surgeon around (in my book) and does a mighty fine job, my scars are downright ug-ugggly! There's no getting around it.

My wonderful husband held me tight in his big strong arms and our ribs touched!!!! Neither of us had been like this since my surgery. We were cheek to cheek, flat chest to flat chest, and I bawled and I bawled and I bawled. I cried buckets and buckets and buckets full of tears. And you already know what happens after that!!! Yep, my nose started going and we had to find the Kleenex and I had to blow my nose and I had to keep blowing it!

You might not believe this, but I'm very private and I don't like to blow my nose in front of anybody. Much less my husband!!! But I had a bucket of Kleenex right beside the tear buckets.

You might be asking yourself.... "Why in the world is she sharing this!!!!!" After all, it was a very private special moment in our life. A part of returning to the new normal. I know some of you will be facing the same thing. I know some of you are facing the same surgery within the next few weeks. I know you're scared. I know you doubt your sexuality. I know some of you have already faced this surgery and in the future, there are going to be more of you facing the same situation. I want you to know you aren't alone!!!

Each of us will take this step in our own way, in our own time. You'll feel very much alone in some of these steps. No one else can enter into the emotions that you go through. We don't expect them. They come out of nowhere it seems. We want to measure how much we're loved. Will we be rejected?? It's hard to look at ourselves sometimes. It's going to go through your head! It just is and there's no stopping it!!!!

My prayer for you my friend, is that your man will love you, like my man loves me.

"Wives, submit yourselves to your husbands, as is fitting to the Lord. Husbands, love your wives and do not be harsh with them." Col 3:18 NIV

"Wives submit yourselves unto your own husbands, as it is fit in the Lord. Husbands, love your wives and be not bitter against them" KJ

"Husbands, love your wives, even as Christ also loved the church, and gave himself for it!" Ephesians 5:25

I am thankful for a God fearing husband who cradles me close to his heart! I pray the same for you!!!

February 22nd, 2014

Thursday, the big 'ole bull came sneaking in with his tail tucked between his legs. I knew he was "skeert" so I just ran and

Back On the Bull (It's anything but normal)

jumped on!!! If you can picture me running up behind the bull and jumping on, then you got the picture! Joe wasn't even with me!!! But, thank goodness Mom and Dad were with me! I "let" dad hold my hand so "he" wouldn't be scared when my port was plugged in! (Isn't that right Nurse Stephanie!) After all they hadn't been with me bull riding yet. I hadn't wanted them to go because I knew it would bother them so much. So of course, I had to be really brave for them which is why I jumped on the bull that way!

I used to high jump in high school so I was really glad I didn't completely jump over the entire bull and land flat on my face!!! I guess that's the advantage of the ageing process. Your jump isn't as high as it used to be.

I think the trip with me helped mom and dad. Mom and I was even playing Kanasta before we left. I was so excited to find out my white blood count was up! Tuesday it was 2 point something. It has to be somewhere between 4 and 11 for me to take chemo. After that big old mean shot I had on Tuesday did its job, my count was over 9 points! Now that is exciting!! Kick up your heels exciting!!

They also backed down my chemo because of my reaction last week and this week was a lot easier. I still don't have my days and nights back in order but we're getting close. I didn't go to sleep until after 4 Friday morning and then not until after 5 on Saturday morning! I may have looked a bit like the deer in the headlights!!

Chemo affects this time: everything taste like chemo! Ugh! Upside of that maybe I won't gain any weight! I've been a little loopy, but not bad. Some might say that's nothing new! I will be skipping chemo this next week so I can get back on my Tuesday schedule. Next scheduled bull ride is March 4th. (Tickets $5 call for reservations!) Thank you all for remembering me and mine in your prayers!!! I love praying for you all!!!

February 24th, 2014

Oh man! That sneaky ole bull came up and butted me from behind!! I went in for my blood test and my white blood count DROPPED to 1.3. Ye' Owl! That's low and I had to take a big ole mean shot! I have to go back in the morning and if it's not high enough I will have to take another shot!!! I was afraid yesterday that it was dropping, but not that low!!!

The Doctor is trying a new thing with me. I am taking Claritin to help with the bone pain from the shot. It really does help a lot! Maybe this will be a medical breakthrough! I have Thing One and Thing Two with me today. Think we'll just lay low and watch cartoons all day!

February 25th, 2014

No bull ride today but my white count is up to 8.8. YEAH!!! I loved getting to see the ladies and gents that work with Joe today! Tonight I am one tired gal. I feel like I could sleep until noon tomorrow!!! My first five hour trip to the office in St. Joe!

February 26th, 2014

Up and at it, had breakfast and dressed to go but the motel clerk said I could keep the room longer. So I get to stay here and rest while Joe is in meetings all morning!

I may as well tell you before Joe does that I got my words all fumbled again yesterday. I was trying to tell him that flour tortillas bother me (because of the chemo). Instead I told him I had a hard time eating the cloth tortillas! Joe was like "The WHAT?" It was pretty funny.

Those of you who know Joe, know that when he laughs he closes his eyes. So we are laughing because I can't get it right and he is driving. If Joe ever ditches the car it will be because he is laughing while he is driving. Oh my!!!

We had supper with one of his clients and some of the staff and it was so sweet it brought tears to my eyes when his client

(Larry Goldberg) did a toast for me! Beer, Fanta soda and sweet tea all clicking together for me! What a great bunch!!! If I have learned anything at all through this journey, it is what an awesome God we have and how wonderful mankind is.

    I had problems with my hair today. For some reason some of the fuzz wanted to stand up instead of lay down. Wonder if some of it's wanting to curl! Ha! Ha! An interesting thought I have since learned. Why does hair curl after chemo? It was explained to me this way. Chemo is so hard on you that the openings where your hair is growing collapses. When your hair tries to grow out it has the same effect as scissors curling ribbon as the hair tries to press out of the opening that has collapsed. Interesting huh!

Chapter 7

Bone-tired, Bald and Water Logged!

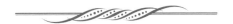

March 1st, 2014

It happens and it's an issue with me. I fall asleep and if something is on my mind, I wake up about 30 minutes later and can't fall back to sleep! I've got to get up and do something. Tonight, I write. It was an interesting conversation to say the least!

This past weekend I ran into an elderly lady that somehow missed that I had been diagnosed. I'm not sure how that happened as I see her quite often. She was shocked to see me and took my arm and said "What has happened to you!!!! Are you sick! What's going on???"

Now I had felt pretty good up until that point but it's true, when someone goes on about how you look and wonders if you are sick you start to feel puny! I was so stunned at her being stunned at how I looked that I just kind of retreated into myself in a manner and watched her face. I had a close up look because she was in my space (or hula hoop as we call it) I tried to lighten the mood and explained I had been diagnosed with cancer in September last year. (Try sometime to lighten a mood with that statement!!!)

She was very shocked. But then she said something that shocked me too. She said… "At least you are wearing a hat! Those bald heads get to me!" WHAT???!!!! I wanted to take my hat off and stuff it in my pocket and say…"Well hats off to you too!" But I didn't.

Instead I found myself not saying anything (at least I don't think I said anything.) Nothing comes to mind and I'm sure if I'd spoke my thoughts out loud my conscious would have bothered me until I apologized. Instead I found myself watching her face and thinking… your elderly and I need to be kind.

What I love about this little lady is her spunk! Do you know that when I was looking for a church to attend; I prayed "God, if it's your will for me to go to New Harmony, please have someone invite me."

Now, I had heard about this church, but I didn't know who attended it; other than three men who I used to work with and hadn't seen in ages. I knew they wouldn't invite me if I did see them! Though it was the testimony of these three men that made me want to attend New Harmony in the first place. All three have since then passed on into eternity.

Two days after my prayer, I happened to run into this lady (I'll call her Ms. Spunk) at Pizza Inn. I stopped by her table and greeted her and she took my hand and said "Karen, why don't you come to church with us sometime." I asked her where she went and she replied "New Harmony!" I replied that I would go! She didn't really think I would but then again, she didn't know what I had prayed just a couple of days earlier. That's been twelve years now! And now you know…. the rest of the story!!

I don't want to just be good…. I want to be Godly!

I don't want to just like you… I want to love you! I don' want to just send you on your way…. I want to walk with you! I don't want to just talk with you…. I want to pray for you! I don't want to just shake your hand…. I want to hug you! I don't want to just listen to you… I want to cry and laugh with you. I want to dance and sing and skip and hop and turn cartwheels. I want to encourage you! When you hurt… I want to feel your pain. When I am old…please be patient with me!! Let us pray….for each other!

March 2, 2014

Recently a friend told me she was taking a marriage bible study class and that she was excited about it! She continued with, 'BUT if they mention the word "submit" I'm out of there!!!"

I've thought about that a lot since then. I was pretty sure the word "submit" was going to be in that bible study!!! Even though I can be a leader in a lot of situations, I really don't have a problem submitting to my (own) husband. Maybe it's because he treats me as "his girl" and "his queen".

Even though I'm very independent on some things. I'm very dependent on others. Like when I get a shot! I like him to hold my hand! I like him to open car doors for me and allow me to walk in a door first.

On the other hand I like to do special things for him. He can do his own laundry, but I like to do it for him. I don't however like to hang up his shirts. I could, but I don't, because he gets such a kick out of making sure his shirts and hangers match. (Mine don't) Our relationship runs pretty smooth.

However today it was a little tense in the house. We didn't share the same opinion on something. My husband felt like I had criticized him. I felt like I was making the project we were working on better. I never once thought the changes I wanted to make were about him or criticizing him. However it was his work I wanted to change even though it was my project that I had asked for some help from him on. I know you married couples have been there before. You know what I'm talking about.

I don't know how it is in your house when there is tension but in our house it gets quiet. Real quiet!!! That's a good thing. It's not always good to say what is going on in your mind until your mind is in the right spot! I picked up my bible and decided to continue a study I had been reading. My marker started at I Peter 3. I begin to read....

"Wives, in the same way submit yourselves to your own husbands so that, if any of them do not believe the word, they may be won over without words by the behavior of their wives!!!"

Whoa! Whoa! Ok now... did Joe change my book mark??? I don't think so. He doesn't know where I'm studying!

Ok... then Karen, back up and take it in. Let's read that over again and apply it to my home. "Karen, in the same way submit yourself to your own husband... (That's Joe) (I'm glad I don't have to submit to anyone else's husband; one is enough!)

So that if any (of them) do not believe the word, (I'm so thankful that my husband believes every word in the bible!) he may be won over without words (Oh my goodness... I have to be quiet and just shut up???) by the behavior (oops...how am I doing today?) of his wife. (That's me) when he see the purity and reverence (oh my... should I reverence him also??? Ok... today would be a good day to make him tea and coconut cream dessert) of your life.

Your beauty should not come from outward adornment, such as elaborate hairstyles (Ok, I've got that one down!!! I run my hands over my fuzzy bald head) and the wearing of gold jewelry or fine clothes. (Sometimes people read that, that we can't wear gold jewelry or fine clothes) I don't believe that's how it reads. Instead that isn't what we should be focused on... instead we should be focused on our inner beauty as it goes on to say in verse 4. Rather, it should be that of your inner self, the unfading beauty of a gentle and quiet spirit (gotta work on that one), which is of great worth in God's sight. (God's watching me!!!??)

My words: If we are depending on the beauty of our youth, or whatever age we are today, it is going to fade! Look in the mirror and see! Look around! But if we are continually working on our inner beauty (attitude, joy, peace, kindness, gentleness, etc.) than that inner beauty won't fade, instead we will be more beautiful every day! (I want to be that girl!!)

Verse 5 goes on to say... For this is the way the holy women of the past who put their hope in God used (have we stopped doing this??) to adorn themselves. They submitted themselves to their own husbands, like Sarah, who obeyed Abraham and called him her lord! (WOW! Joe would fall on the ground laughing if I called him lord! However.... He would love for me to treat him as one! I can do that with love and joy!!!

It continues... You are her daughters if you do what is right and do not give way to fear! FEAR??? What are they talking about??? I trace the reference... Genesis 18 verse 12. "So Sarah laughed to herself as she thought, "After I am worn out and my lord is old, will I now have this pleasure?" hummmmm... You know the story! God had promised Abraham a child in his old age! Instead of relying on God's word and her husband's relationship with God. Sarah took things into her own hands and made a mess of things! She actually ran her husband off to have a child with another woman!!

Now any of us women are thinking we would never do that!!! But we see it happen all the time, don't we!!! Our relationship with our husbands can be "Come here...come here...come here...no... get away...get away...get away!" or "I love you... here...eat these mud pies!" We love, but we don't respect. The one thing God tells us to give our husbands!!! (Respect)

I often hear couples say "Marriage is hard!" It doesn't have to be. You can have hard days...but marriage in itself can be easy. When we line our marriage up with God's word, marriage becomes easy.

The bible says we women are to submit to our own husbands and why and how. That's usually questions a woman wants to know...to who? How come and ok...how do I do that? That's our part. The man also has a part. We women of course don't like to let them off the hook, do we? Maybe I can get Joe to comment on that part that comes right after we're told to submit. (1 Peter 3 V 7) He only has one verse! There was six verses for the women.

Ladies...you may or may not know this... but there is power in submitting!!!! Sarah did (later) submit and she did have pleasure and received that child in her old age! WOW! Her husband still desired her in her old age!!!! Makes old age not seem so bad doesn't it!! Guess I'd better get up from here and go work on that coconut dessert!!!

March 3rd, 2014

Oh man, I had to take a shot today to get my white blood count up so I'll be ready for chemo tomorrow. I wasn't prepared to look the bull in the eye but I will be tomorrow. I'm not too sure but I'm thinking that shot was a bull ride in disguise. Please don't tell me there is more than one bull in that room!! Dreading.........

March 4th, 2014

WOW! What a sendoff at the chemo room today!!! Joe had to work and wasn't able to go with me! (Well...somebody has to pay these DR and Lab bills) My wonderful friend Diane Ross from Nebraska came down to be with me a few days while Joe works. She went with me to chemo to drive me home. Nobody wants to be on the road with me driving after chemo. I can hardly walk a straight line, much less get behind the wheel of a vehicle!!!

We arrived at the Bond Clinic and as predicted my baby sister is ALWAYS there with a homemade card for me!! I love her to the moon and back! You should see her beautiful cards! That gal has talent!!! With her to surprise me was my two handsome, wonderful, precious nephews!! (Jacob and Brandon!) Now there's two guys who know how to give an aunt a hug!! Since I am their only aunt, I get to be their favorite aunt!!! How cool is that!!

All this love and picture takin' in the waiting room, plus all of your encouragement and prayers made me walk in there with a purpose. Sucker punch that bull!! I slumped my shoulders over... got my 'I'm gonna get cha' stance on.... (Kind of looked like an ape going forward) and stomped in to look that ole bull right in the eye!!

I knew he was going to do it! My back up man had to work and 'ole bull must have known he wasn't there to hold my hand... so he looked back at me, square in the eye!!! What he didn't know... was I had plan "B" with me. Diane already knew

I had chicken liver for guts so she reached over and held my hand while I got my port plugged in and the bull blinked first during our stare down!!! That means... I won!!!! La...la..la...la..la!!!

It's day one and as long as these steroids are working, I'm feeling mighty fine!! It's midnight and I'm thinking, "Oh sleep wherefore art thou!" Fried taters, cornbread, brown beans and salad for supper and I got to help cook and clean up! I'm not going to mention that I fell asleep twice during conversations earlier. Some things are just better left unsaid.

Thank you all for your prayers!! You may not know how much I count on them and how beautiful you all are to me!! I love you each and am praying blessings right back on each of you! Thank you and I thank God for hearing all of our prayers and for his blessings being poured out on each of us!! He loves YOU and so do I!!!

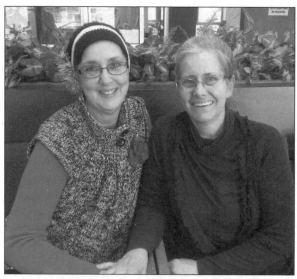

My longtime friend Diane Ross came all the way from Nebraska to help and spend time with me.

March 9th, 2014

Thing One and Thing Two were so excited to get to be at our house today. They wanted a tea party as soon as they came in. Thing Two ALWAYS asks where Poppy Joe is as soon as she walks in the door. I told her. "He's working in at the office (in town)" She thought I meant his office here at the house. She took off running down the hall to see her beloved Poppy Joe. She came back running, telling me "You'd better check it out Nana, he's not in his office!"

Since my energy was low, I suggested a kid's movie for them. We generally don't turn on a movie unless it's nap time and the girls pile on me and fall asleep about five minutes into the move. However, they were too excited and Thing One said to me, "Thing Two has already had her N...A...P!"" Thing two replied, "I don't want a N...A...P!"

March 10th, 2014

Bull riding today!!! Oh why can't I fall asleep!!!!!

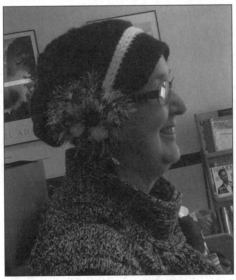

One of my many fun hats!

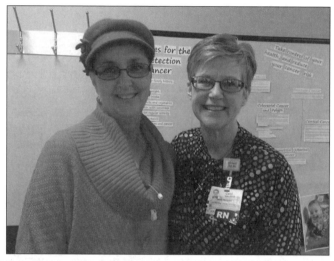

My Nurse Navigator Carol Walters. She walks you through all of your steps. You're in good hands with Carol!!

March 11th 2014

It seems like lately, as the journey continues, I've just been feeling so often that it's a long journey. I find myself saying over and over that I'm so tired of this and ready to get on with my life. It's kind of like... I'm not really here right now. But it's really not like that at all. Chemo brain or not I'm all here in the moment. I'm not really sure where I am. Have I met the half way point or not? All I know is I'm learning one day at a time. It seems like I learn that one over and over. On one side it's a good lesson to learn. On the other side, I'm impatient. So what's it like to be seven months into the journey and about four more months to go. WOW!!! I'm over half way!!! Who can kick as high as a door post? The top of the door.... no cheating!!!

    I am so looking forward to my celebration party!!! Don't forget to save the date. Yeah... I know, but I'll post it as soon as I know when it is!! However today, the journey is long.

    Here's what I'm tired of; "All of it." But let's break it down. I'm tired of short hair! It's coming in all colors!! Right now it's sparkly on top and black on the sides. Your guess is as good as mine, but I'm not saying the other word for sparkly, but I hope I don't look like a skunk with black eyebrows!!! Just saying!!!

I watched my dad the other day. Ever notice how a man stretches out and rubs his tummy after a good meal??? We women never do that!!! As I looked at my dad I thought.... "Oh NO! Now I'm built like my dad, I could do that!" I've got his long legs, tummy. His flat chest. He has more hair than me. I even have a lot of his personality. I could be his son!!! YIKES!! Please stop me if you see me rubbing my tummy!

I'm tired of clothes that don't fit!! The other day I went shopping with some friends. We ended up at dress barn where $79 tops were marked down to $10!! Yeah.... better run! You can come back and finish this later!!! I took a handful to the dressing room and ended up in tears! I can't wear anything with darts!! That includes jackets!!! My size DRAPES over my shoulder like a too big sack! I go to a smaller size and it's too short. I'm tired of that already!!!

I'm tired of chemo brain!!! I mean, I get ready to say something and oh! What was it I was saying????? I'm tired of shots, and being light headed and numb toes! I'm tired of drinking, water...water...water...water....water. I'm tired of getting up in the middle of the night to go to the bathroom four times! I'm tired of not being able to fall asleep. I'm tired of falling asleep in the middle of conversations.

I'm tired of needing help and feeling lazy when I get it. I'm tired of not being able to focus. I'm tired of my weight going up and down like a yo yo! I'm very tired of not being able to have Thing One and Thing Two at my house because I'm tired. I'm tired of getting tired when I go grocery shopping and having to lean on the buggy all the way back to the car. I'm tired of you seeing me as tired.

I am tired of falling asleep in the middle of praying for you! I am tired of not being able to eat because food taste like chemo. I'm tired of chemo and bandages that stick when you pull them off! I am tired of chemo streaks on my finger nails! I'm tired of my toe nails and finger nails falling off! Did you know chemo does that to you?

STOP!! STOP!! STOP IT!! This being tired "ain't a movin" me!!!! Put some rhythm in your rhyme and some beat in your music girl!!!! I am thankful...for God, who holds my hand through it all! I am thankful for family who is always standing by me! For friends who have not left my side! Who have run the sweeper, dusted furniture, mopped floors, and brought meals.

I am thankful for every phone call just calling to check. For the wonderful cards and every word of encouragement! I'm thankful for every hug! I'm thankful for the ones who have brought us firewood! For hoodies and for flowers! For everyone who has gone to chemo with me and for those who have asked to go but haven't had a turn yet! I'm thankful you WANT to go with me! I'm thankful for wonderful DR's and for nurses who go beyond the call of duty!

I'm thankful for everyone who has told me I wear no hair beautifully!!! You've helped me through many a bad no hair day! I'm thankful for gifts of blankets, socks, pajamas, books, jewelry, pillowcases, meals, desserts, potato soup, bath oils, scarves, hats, quilts and knitted shawls. I'm thankful for pictures, bracelets, posters, pears, apples, Christmas ornaments, beautiful scarves and inspirational books, homemade cookies and unexpected visits and private messages!!!

I'm thankful for tea parties and surprise parties and for those of you who know a girl can't make it far without chocolate! I'm thankful for unexpected private gifts, for stuffed peppers and pie! I'm thankful for magazines and snacks and book bags! I'm thankful for those who have showed up at surgery time and PET scan time and waited patiently during long days and anxious moments. For showing up when I was too sick to be left by myself. I'm thankful for patient clients and customers. I'm thankful for prayers from family, friends and strangers!!!

I'm thankful for the new friends I have made and for those I haven't met yet!! I'm thankful for old friends who have stayed by my side! For every word of encouragement and support. I'm thankful for everyone who has not grown weary of this journey!

Bone-tired, Bald and Water Logged!

I cannot begin to list everything or everyone!! I am thankful for YOU and your prayers! I'm thankful I can pray for you!

I am thankful for parents who worry about me every day because they love me. For biscuits and gravy and cornbread and brown beans! I'm thankful for a sister who changed her Monday off to a Tuesday so she could drop by and bring me a homemade card at every chemo visit! For her taking pictures and posting for me! I'm thankful for nieces and nephews who have surprised me with visits and hugs!!! I'm thankful for sister-in-laws who come to help (SEVEN weeks) and who call to check or just to visit. I'm thankful for the support of brother-in-laws and pats on the back!

I'm thankful for my beautiful grandkids who call me and tell me they love me! I'm thankful for grand-girls who rub my head and say... "I love you bald head"! I'm thankful for every time they say "I love you Nana!" even if it's fifteen times in twenty minutes!!! I'm thankful for my three wonderful sons who constantly call and check on me or contact me on chat when they see me on Facebook.

I am thankful for a husband who can cook and clean! Who holds me when I cry and kisses my bald head when my hair falls out and tells me I'm cute and beautiful even when I'm not crying over my figure or an outfit that doesn't fit. I'm thankful for his support and patience and his assurance that he'll always be here for me! I'm thankful for his hugs and for his reaching for my hand constantly! I'm thankful for his prayers over me! I'm thankful he's a godly man. I'm thankful for his humor!

I'm thankful for a God in heaven who sees all! I'm thankful that I know HIM! I'm thankful for rainbows and whispers in the night! I'm thankful God answers prayers! I'm thankful for Jeremiah 29:11 and Psalms 34:17-22 and Psalm 118:17 & 18. I'm thankful for this journey and that, this too shall pass.

Lord, help me to learn the lesson in this test. Help me to lift my feet above the pebbles that make me stumble! Help me to show your glory through this journey, to remember this is your battle and I'm only an instrument in your hand. Thank you for holding me in the palm of your hand for not letting me go when my faith has been weak. I ask you to pour your blessings out on each who have prayed for or encouraged me in any way! Family and friends and strangers alike! Bless even those who have prayed for me that I don't even know about! Abundantly bless the little children who have prayed for me and those little kids who have sent me little cards and prayed for me in their Sunday school classes! I am humbled by these little ones that I don't even know! Lord bless them and keep them safe every day of their lives!

I am humbled by the love and care shown to Joe and me by family, friends and strangers. Lord bless each one and their families!! I am especially humbled by your gifting your son to a lost world that we might know YOU and be saved! Thank you Lord for your greatest gift of all! We praise your name and give you all the glory! In Jesus name we ask these things in faith of you and your word. Amen

March 16th, 2014

In the beginning there were three of us sisters. Lynn, Karen and Jill. We lost our beloved Lynn 12 years ago to ovarian cancer. She only lived a couple of weeks after finding out she had ovarian cancer and it was a desperate hard time. Because of losing our Lynn, it's been especially hard on my family that I was diagnosed with breast cancer.

My baby sister Jill has not left my side. She has been helping me with this water drinking deal that I have to do. I have to drink 5 bottles of water every day. Now, I'm a sipper and not a drinker. In my "regular life", I would normally drink only two or three bottles. I can make a bottle last a half a day. Jill has decided to help me with the drinking by drinking five bottles a day too. Jill is very talented and writes poetry. Here's her poem for me concerning the five bottles of water we have to drink a day!

To my sister, Karen, Love Jill Marie Neugebauer

Five bottles of water doesn't seem like a lot
And in 24 hours, it's probably not!
But 8 of those hours, I much prefer sleep
Instead of hourly, "taking a leak"!

But I promised my sister
we would both "drink together"
Hoping that this
would make her feel better!

Now we're BOTH water-logged
and we're starting to waddle
as we grimace & groan...
And grab our next bottle.

Every 15 minutes
it's 5 gulps down...
Then grab another bottle
and go another round!

Our bellies are rounded
and our brains cannot think...
Eyes starting to water
But still we must drink!

Around 8pm, I grab my 5th bottle.
I try to down it by 10.
But before I know it, I'm ready to throw it...
'Cause I can't fit anymore in!

Soon this will be over
My Sis will be well!
With laughter & love
new stories we'll tell.

We'll dance in the rain,
We'll shop 'til we drop...
But instead of just water
I think we'll drink "POP"!!

I'd love to write more
but I really must "GO"...
After all, you must realize
I'm full of H2O!!!!!!!!!!!!

March 17th, 2014

The bull and I have been going around in circles the past few days. He acts friendly but I'm not about to turn my back on him!! My blood count has dropped to what they call a "Panic Low' so I'm not sure I'll be able for chemo tomorrow. I had to take another one of those mean shots today!!! I'm not liking this one little bit!!! Thank you for your prayers!!! I love you all bunches and am praying for you too!!!   Happy 61st anniversary to my parents!

March 18th, 2014

I should be sleeping… and you should be too… instead I try to sneak out of bed and head to my computer. I try not to wake my sleeping husband as I slip from the warm bed. I hope he doesn't hear the side of the bed squeak. I've learned which floor boards to not step on and make it all the way to the living room without a sound. I close the bedroom door and it squeaks. I hold my breath… Joe doesn't move. I let it squeak again as I completely shut it so I can turn the light on and not disturb him. It's not that I wouldn't welcome his company tonight. He just needs his rest since it's been a rough few days. We have another big day ahead of us. After all… it's another saddle up the bull riding day.

I'm often asked about that bull ride. After all when they saddle up those bulls in the chemo room, they all look calm.

I have never seen anyone saddle up and not have a calm exterior about them. I'm probably the biggest chicken liver in the room, but how does one describe the thunder that can roll through their veins??? How do you describe being so wide awake and wanting to sleep at the same time.

Tonight it's the shot I get to make me build white blood cells that is the bull ride. I can't even describe it but even though I fell asleep when I first went to bed, I wake myself up with the words, "mercy, mercy, please Lord have mercy". There really are no words to describe how these shots can make you feel. And... I'm one of the lucky ones!

Some people are very sick and have tons of pain. My pain is just enough to make me miserable. Just enough that I can't lay still. Just enough that, I start rubbing my arms... rubbing my legs... ru*bbing my bald head. I just want to sleep!!! To rest!!! I know I'm going to need my energy tomorrow to get through another needle stabbing.* I continue to rub my arms and legs, my back and squeeze my shoulders trying to get myself to relax and I realize, I'm crying. I'm too tired and I'm feeling desperate.

I'm pretty sure with how I'm feeling that I'm not going to have chemo tomorrow. After all this bull tonight is about all I can handle. Quite frankly... I'm scared spitless of that bull tomorrow. I'm not always afraid of him, well... I am a little, but not like tonight when I'm even too tired to look him eyeball to eyeball. My tears flow and I know there's only one way out of this mess! I begin to rub my fuzzy bald head and pray.

I pray your name and I go right on down the street and keep praying... through our town, in our church, the chiropractors, the post office and each of the business' in town...into the hospital and for the DR and nurses... I name you one by one. I hop over to Florida and begin my cousin list which takes me all the way up the eastern states, and into West Virginia and Ohio While I'm there I get my Michigan friends and classmates in Ohio and Joe's family, aunts and uncles nieces and nephews. There's a whole group in Ohio that I don't even know that keep cheering me on. I pray for those who have had or have cancer on my list and their families. God and I have an understanding. When I mention your name, not only do I want you covered, but I want your family covered too.

I grab more Kleenex and keep rubbing my head and my back. I pray for my face book friend in Australia and for friends who are out of the country traveling. I hop over to the western part of the states and cover friends and family and strangers alike. We take on the Midwest including Tennessee and Alabama and the big ole state of Texas. I can tell I'm calming down.

I pray for those in the chemo room and for my children and grandchildren, for my parents and for Joe, for our sisters and families. I pray for our pastor and his wife and every name I can think of in the church. I pray for the likes and comments on face book. For those who are struggling and just had surgery. I pray for my son's classmates who have sent me messages and encouragement. For ex's in the family that took part of my heart. I pray for strangers that I don't know who have sent me messages and encouragement.

I thank God every night isn't like tonight…some nights I can't remember ten names. Sometimes… If I were counting, it might be 100 names. Tonight we're marching up and down the streets praying for you because it gives me strength and encourages me to do so. Also because I love you bunches.

My heart rest. Even though I don't think I'll pass the bull test tomorrow, I do feel more relaxed, though my body still throbs. You might wonder why I'm sharing this with you… but as the tears ran down my cheeks and my hands went over my fuzzy bald head…and your name tumbled off my lips; it was like I had to share how important you are in this journey with me. You help me take my mind off of me. Thank you for walking along beside me. Thank you for not growing weary.

If this pain doesn't ease… I'm going to have to start all over. Which state should I start with first this time………

Go on out to pasture old bull... I'm not riding you today!! Special thanks today to my Joe, my sister, your prayers, the receptionist, nurses and DR Nevils who helped me through this morning. I love you each!!! Go on get... Bull... don't look at me like that!!! Next week I'll whip you once again!!!

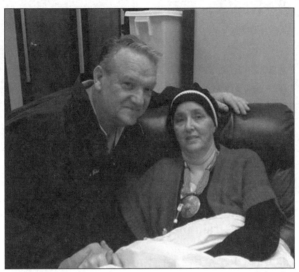

This week didn't start out so good. Bladder infection And high dose of the shot yesterday! Tremendous pain!

March 21st, 2014

My kind of Friday!! Date with my hubby for lunch. Then off I headed with friends to the Rolla Home Show!!! Girls' night out at Fat Cats. (Paddle auction) No chemo this week. Woooo Hoooo!! A day to kick up my heels a bit. Wondering if I could get by with wearing a crown instead of a hat this beautiful day! I can't seem to just get a flower to stick!

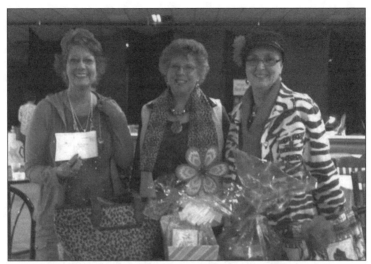
Colleen Hills, Loretta Phelps and me with our loot from the quarter auction.

Old Bull may look mean, tough and ugly, but I have full intentions of riding him again Tuesday! Lord, help me keep my courage up and whip this beast!!! My legs are longer than his; but he's got four!!!

March 25th, 2014

I was ready to saddle up, but the bull ran off! This is the second time we've tried to do week seven!!

DR Nevils explained there will be no bull ride this week. Due to low numbers and wanting me to complete my antibiotics. We're not taking any risks! Thank you DR Nevils for your good care!

I have to tell you.... 'Ole Bull was chicken this week! I may have to find another picture of him!!! I went in all ready to jump on him but DR Nevils made the decision for me to not saddle up, so I got another week off. I couldn't believe how fast those four little fat legs ran from me!! Made me giggle!!!

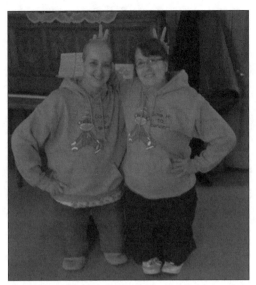

Cancer really does cost an arm and a leg! It's wearing us down! Jill and I add a little humor to the situation!

Tee shirt...jeans....and tennis shoes! I do believe there are days I could pass for my father's son! I don't like that at all!!!

March 31st, 2014

UGH.... trying to purge my closet of things that no longer fit!!! I like that...nope...doesn't fit! How about this... nope can't keep it on my shoulders... how about this....nope... grrrrr Change in schedule this week. Blood work on Tues. Expect chemo on Wed. Working on my prayer wall names, still working on taxes!!!

Old Bull looks like a mean beast and he is! He actually scares the heebie jeebies out of me!!! After a two week break, I plan to hop on and ride him again on Wednesday. Gotta make it to the half way point! You would think a person would get used to this, but I don't think anybody gets used to chemo running through their veins. Nope! Ya just don't. Thank you for continuing to pray for me! I am still praying for you!

Chapter 8

Happy Birthday to Me!
39 Plus Tax and Shipping

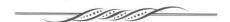

April 1st, 2014

It was a good day! I did more today than I've done in a LONG time! Ran the sweeper, mopped the floors, changed sheets, cleaned the bathrooms, the kitchen, cooked, cleaned up and worked on changing out my closet (though I'm not near done on that!) Yes it was a very good day indeed!!!

April 2nd, 2014

For sure this time... no April Fooling! I finally got to do week 7. For real!!
    Halfway point crossed! Thanks Karen Stephens for helping me saddle up the bull this week!

April 4th, 2014

I'm so excited to have crossed the center line!!! After trying three times...I managed to hop back on that bull!! I'm now halfway through my chemo treatments!! Let's see... eyelashes are falling out again...Hair is growing..."some" ... fingernails are growing off!!!

It's really weird. Did you know that when you take chemo the lines in your fingernails go crossways? When you have toxins in your body like this instead of the ridges going up and down, they start showing up sideways and make lines like a growth line on a tree. I have to be very careful with my nails now because as they grow off, if they are hit just right can really hurt and could break off. It looks like fake nails grown out too far. I am no longer vain!!! Mercy! I have been stripped of any vanity I may have or may not have had in the past!!! Pride be gone... is gone!!! I'm still having to drink 5 - 6 bottles of water a day.

Today Judy Thompson from the Methodist Church in Salem, came out and brought me the sweetest gift from her church!! It's a prayer blanket. Every knot tied represents an individual prayer for ME!!! When someone prayed for ME (yes it has my name on it) they placed their hand on the blanket and then tied a knot. Once all of the knots were tied (and there is a bunch of them) she brought me the blanket. It's beautiful and I appreciate it very much. More than anything I appreciate the prayers!!!! What a gift!!!! Thank you to each of you who participated in this!

April 7th, 2014

I'm beginning to think I'm on vacation. Either that or 'Ole Bull has been put out to pasture! Let's see... I've been lying around soaking up the sun in front of my bay window. That's about as close to a vacation as we're going to get for a while! It looks like I'm going to get another week "off" this week. NO chemo tomorrow!!!! I would cheer but that means it just takes longer until my celebration party! I am ready to be done with this and party!!! Who is with me?

April 9th, 2014

Weary....just plum weary of all of this!! How can one be so weary when the sun is shining through the window like it is today? I must need a nap and an attitude adjustment!

When I receive messages of your stories, I'm reminded how unfair life can be at times. How thankful I am to each of you who have encouraged me and especially to those who have struggled this cancer journey yourself and shared your incredible stories with me. I love you each and continue to pray for you!!!

@Kandie Stock I cannot believe we didn't get pictures last night for my journal and Facebook journal! So, can you and Paul please go back to RED ROBIN YUMMMMM and order the 13 Onion Ring Stack, then eat a hamburger (& fries) and order the MONSTER MOUNTAIN of a dessert AGAIN..... And take pictures this time!!!!

April 10th, 2014

Fact One: Sometimes I ponder my words. I roll them around in my mind carefully and then I voice my thoughts. Other times I even surprise me with what comes out and my hand flies to my mouth. This happens way too often.

Fact Two: I'm not often moody. Something usually has ticked me off if I am moody.

Fact Three: I am bald! I know it. You know it. Everyone who sees me knows it! So tonight I have pondered some of my words. Enough so that I have had to get out of bed and head to my computer. Others I have not pondered. I'll leave you to guess which is which!!

I am also ticked off. That means I am moody. I'm hitting just about any place on the scale. Your guess is as good as mine! It all has to do with being bald! Oh what I'd do to have my long hair back! NOW! Not last month... not next fall... NOW! My hair now might be 1/4 inch long. I'm as fuzzy as a new puppy! My hair is betraying me though. It went out one color and is coming in another color. I'm not pleased!

My mother told me the other day that I'm rockin' being bald! That's pretty good coming from my mother who hasn't been known to throw that many compliments my way. She was always afraid I'd get the big head. I did anyway; oh well.

None of that has anything to do with my being ticked off and moody though!

My experience yesterday caused it. I'm a friendly sort of gal! I look you in the eye and what you see is what you get! I love to give you a smile and hope I made your day go a bit smoother for it! I want to encourage you and encourage you to get in the race and run, I want YOU at the party! I want to be a bright spot in your day! I want you to know that even if nobody else cares; I do.

I am also a people observer. Yesterday we were out of town at a hospital where my brother-in-law was having back surgery. We had to walk up long hallways several times a day and we passed many, many people. I love people!!

I had removed my "bad hair day" hat and had decided to just not wear it. Have you ever tried to wear a hat all day!!! I knew a lot of the people were working hard and a lot were stressed because of loved ones at the hospital etc. So I began smiling at each one I passed and giving them a nod. I'm sure I passed between 30 - 50 people, smiling and nodding during the course of the day. Only one lady smiled back at me. Everyone else looked at me in a sort of shocked look and then pretended they hadn't seen me! Staring straight ahead!

I kept thinking... "But mama says I rock this look!" I began to believe "mama was wrong"! It became a game to me and I kept smiling and nodding. Observing each response. At the end of the day I'd received one smile back! It hurt my feelings, ticked me off and I got moody! I felt like a freak and invisible! Moody makes me weepy!

Tonight as I was praying (I started east of town tonight) I began to think of all of you and how you have cheered me on and supported me! I began to wonder why strangers I don't even know could have had such an effect on my mood. And then I looked for what I could learn from this experience because I don't want to miss any lessons that I'm supposed to learn from this journey.

I wondered how many times have I failed to acknowledge someone with a disability or because I was uncomfortable with the situation they were in. How many times have I turned my eyes because I didn't know what to say or what not to say? How many times have I looked at YOU and seen your burden and yet turned my eyes away. How many times could I have just smiled and given you a nod to let you know you're not alone and yet I adverted my eyes and kept on rolling? How many times have I been so wrapped up in myself... and my own thoughts that I've failed to reach out to someone who had a hand out for help?

As always when I start feeling bad about me and my situation I start praying for you! Goodness! How I've prayed for you these past eight months!!! But God says... "It's not all about me" anyway! So I'm going to keep on rockin' it and I'm going to keep on smiling! I did make one person's moment! She smiled back!!! I don't know, maybe I had broccoli in my teeth. Non-the-less, she still smiled and made my day!

April 12th, 2014

WOW! I was quiet amazed at all of your responses both here and on my personal Facebook page concerning my smile experiment the other day. Thank you to each of you and to those who personal messaged and called me!! You know what I like so much about this way of communicating and sharing! It's YOU!!! You all are so quick to encourage and pray!!! You are on here, not only encouraging me, but each other. That is awesome!!

I love hearing everyone's opinions and deep thoughts!!! I love hearing how you encourage each other by reading each other's post. You are blessing one another abundantly!!! I'm in awe!!

This week looks promising! After missing chemo last week, and a new medication, I'm feeling like a new person. Just don't ask me to get up!!!

I have a DR appointment Monday to check on the bull to see if he's going to be willing for a ridin' this week. I'm not expecting him to tuck tail and run; but you never know. To be such a bully, (no pun intended) he can sure turn chicken and run sometimes. We do need to get these next six treatments done with. I'm appreciating your prayers and pray God will pour out his blessings on YOU abundantly!!

Thank you Michele Gragert-Vaughn for going the 10 Mile AVON walk for me!! What a special gift! I feel honored!!

April 14th, 2014

Heading up to see if the Bull is ready for riding. If I get to ride this week; next week will be a five fingers week! Dreading it but wanting it over with!! Thank you for your prayers! Praying blessings on you too!!!

April 17th, 2014

Seriously.... I think I winded that bull when I hopped on this time! I know it winded me!!! I've been either WIDE awake or SOUND asleep! No in-betweens!! It's the first time that I've swollen so much from the steroids that I'm not able to wear my rings! Three trips a week to the clinic is getting "tedious"!!! It's bedtime for me. Thank you all for praying so faithfully for me!!! I appreciate it more than you'll ever know!!! Joe and I continue to pray for each of you!!

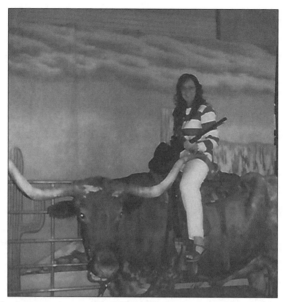

See! I really can get on a bull!! Just thought you'd like to see this! Taken in Texas when I had hair!!! Yes he is real and very much alive!!

April 18th, 2014

Thank you Sarah Parks for going with me to chemo! I hope everything I said made "perfect sense". I love you girlfriend and so appreciate you!!

Little Brianna "Sweet Bug"!! I am praying for you!!! Brianna is 8 years old and has Leukemia. Please join me in praying for her!!

April 20th, 2014

I loved waking up today to the sun shining through the windows!!! It's just a reminder to me that our Lord rose! I have enjoyed reading all of the post today and how happy and cheerful all have been. If you listen to the news, you might think Christianity is falling apart. But talk to your neighbor and friends and family and you'll see that it's alive and well! This year I have been more grateful than ever! As God has answered your prayers and mine on so many issues, I've watched our faith increase!!! Call me grateful!!!   Happy Easter everyone!

April 21st, 2014

Well that didn't quite go as planned!!! All of my counts were good! That's good! NO shot today! That's good!!! BUT... I caught a virus. NOT good!! Been one sick gal! Not good! No bull ride tomorrow!! Just sleeping and on a liquid diet for the next 24 hours!! Feeling bummed out!!!

April 26th, 2014

WOW! Today and yesterday have been a celebration of both life and death!! I want to honor my Uncle Junior Phillips first in his celebration of death today. He was an ornery uncle! At a family reunion, he would most likely be the one in the center of attention with the kids and you could always bet somebody was going to get wet! He had a giggle when he laughed. He loved country music and playing the guitar. He picked on everyone! Yes... we'll miss him as he dances down those streets of gold!!!

Yesterday for me, was my birthday! For me it wasn't about presents and cake (even though I appreciated every gift and both of the cakes. (one from my dad and one from my nephew Jacob!) I was just happy to be alive!

I want to thank EVERY ONE of you for your birthday wishes, e-cards, birthday cards, special notes & gifts! I have always loved my birthday "month" but I have never before felt the excitement about being alive as I did this birthday! Let me share my day with you!

My wonderful hubby took me out for breakfast and announced to everyone that it was my birthday! Everyone in the restaurant wished me happy birthday of course. I went skipping out the door to get my driver's license renewed. I put my wig on before going in. I just don't have enough hair yet to be able to wear it comfortably and it's hot! Truth is, I hate wearing a wig and feel "fake" in it. It just isn't me!!

I passed my sign test and ABC test with flying colors. I paid my fee for my new license and took my wig off and put my hat on. The lady looked at me and said "We haven't taken your picture yet!!!" She should have taken it then! I had such a stunned look on my face! It was a hoot!! The only reason I wore the wig in the first place was because I didn't want my picture on my license to be bald for several years!

I headed to Rolla. Several friends had contacted me this week and said if I was able they'd like to take me to lunch for my birthday. I decided to tell each one who asked... "Yes, I'd go!" I of course was asked where I wanted to go and so as each asked I told them where I wanted to go. Each thought they were the only one eating with me!!! I got to the restaurant early and secured a table for all of us. It was an awesome party! After all... I couldn't just accept one invitation could I?? Some knew each other, some were related and some made brand new friends!! Fun huh!!!

Not long after lunch I had to go rest and take a nap. (Not fun, but after all... the three nine numbers (39) did get bigger this year) Happy 58th birthday to me!! Better known in our family as 39 plus tax and shipping! Family gathered at Mom and Dad's for my family birthday party. When we drove in the driveway at home there before my eyes... my wonderful hubby had planted flowers just for me!!! What a guy!!!!

I just want to thank everyone for helping me celebrate my life this year!!! I certainly had a kick up your heels sort of day! I am blessed beyond what I have ever imagined. I thank God for each of you and continue to pray for you!!! Hug your loved ones! You never know if you'll be celebrating life or death. Love one another and make each day special!!!

April 30th, 2014

I'm still riding the bull. He's knocked me around a bit. When I walked in to get plugged in.... (What's wrong with this picture?) I'd rather have one of those mechanical bulls that plug in where I could drop a quarter in and unplug him if I wanted!!

Those were the good old days!! A quarter doesn't get you much now days though! Especially in the medical field!! Anyway, I've already strayed from my point!

You might think the bull ride only last while at the clinic However it's about a three/four day ride. That bull thunders through my veins in a way I can hardly explain! It's like swimming under water and even though you might tell me what I say makes sense, I feel like nothing makes sense and I'm afraid what I say doesn't sound connected. I'm not sure if my brain is jumping around from thought to thought too fast or if it's completely stopped.

I walk in there feeling pretty good, like I can conquer a mountain only to walk out of there not being able to walk a straight line! I think the worse part of my time there is seeing so many be able to just conk out and take a nap. I am so sleepy from the medicine and yet my body wants to jerk so much I can't relax and fall asleep.

Exhaustion generally hits me on the way home and I sleep all afternoon. That makes it hard to get to bed on time. I did however manage to get about three hours of sleep from midnight until three this morning. I lay there trying to go back to sleep (not happening) and trying not to toss and wake Joe. (Lack of sleep does not bode well with him)

Lying in bed leads to praying! I hope you are feeling extra blessed today! I've been rattling off your names before the Lord! I so love praying for each of you! I'm still working on my prayer wall and hope to have it at my celebration party sometime this summer. The names just keep getting longer and longer and I want to put them in alphabetical order. You have no idea how much your prayers mean to me. I think of you every day and appreciate each of you! I am well aware that I've been doing so well because you have not ceased to remember me and have prayed so diligently for me. I want to be as diligent in praying for you!!! I am impressed and so appreciate and love each of you. Thank you for praying!!!

This past week was like a roller coaster ride and wouldn't you know it, my seat was shaped like a bull!!! One moment I was up and so excited about being alive for my birthday! Not that I have doubted for a moment (that I wouldn't be). I am just so thankful for LIFE! The next moment I was discouraged because I'd hardly crossed the half way point {with chemo} when I should have crossed the finish line last week! I thought I'd never get to hold up just five fingers for my picture!!

Chemo this time has taken more hair. It's wiped out my eye lashes and not only is that creepy, it's downright uncomfortable! Who would have thought?

Thing One is so excited that I have hair growing. That's a sign to her that I'm getting better! However I dread it when she realizes that it's thinning again!!! Every week when I see her, she rubs my head and says..."Your hair is growing Nana!" She does it like she's trying to encourage me!! So sweet!

Yesterday she grabbed my hat off, put it on her head, rubbed my hair and said again. "Your hair is growing Nana!" Then she squinted up her little face and popped her eyes like she does and said "I think it's coming in gray!" Then to make me feel "not alone" she said "My Yaw Yaw" has gray hair too!" That's her other grandpa. I said "Oh! So do you like gray hair?" She said... "No." Hum... the honesty of a little child. I said... "Well maybe I'll just have to change its color but you do know gray hair means you're wise!" The wisdom part went right over her head (I saw it go) and she answered "YES! Make it the color it used to be BROWN!" I sure do love that girl!!

Chapter 9

Just Cleaning Up My Plate!

May 2nd, 2014

We decided today that instead of my hat saying "Bad Hair Day", it might have been better to say "Moody" day! I had a hard time dragging myself out of bed this morning, but had to get up since I had a DR appointment to see if I needed a shot.

I did! UGH!! I do not like those shots. My blood count was down again from chemo this week. Just knowing I should have been done with the chemo and I'm not makes me weepy.

When you have eye lashes, your tears can lie gently on your lashes and roll down your cheeks in a feminine manner. All girls know this. When you don't have eyelashes, they just dump down your cheeks or roll out the sides of your eyes. Makes a gal moody not to be able to bat eye lashes when needed. Joe was with me today, I needed my eyelashes!

Breakfast, lunch and supper all taste like cardboard flavored food! Ever chew on cardboard? It doesn't matter what color it is, it's all the same!

I had a good report from my surgeon! That's exciting! There's nothing quite like a good report! I'm healing really well. I am however, not going to be able to run the sweeper and do some of the things I thought I was going to be able to do and have been trying to do. I didn't realize how much I really do like to clean house and organize things until... oh well... where's that ole "Moody" hat anyway. I'm thinking I now need some chocolate (lots of it) and I'm going to have to pray for you real hard tonight!! Do you ever get moody and need a hat?

May 4th, 2014

Something has been on my mind for quite some time and I've wanted to mention it to you. You all know that October is Breast Cancer awareness month. So many of you go in October to get your mammogram. That's good. I want to suggest to you that you go earlier in the year. Here's why. You have a deductible with your insurance. You also have a percentage you have to pay on top of that, be it 20% or 30% or whatever it is. It can all add up.

My experience was I was diagnosed in September. I had my deductible to reach and my percentage. Our insurance changed the first of December so I had a new deductible and percentage with a new company. In January, it all starts over and again and you have to reach your deductible and percentage again. I hope you are following my train of thought here. Had I gone in January last year or at least earlier in the year, I wouldn't have it hit so high. Of course in January, I didn't know I had cancer! However my treatments will take about a year all told by the time I'm finished. This does not include follow up etc. What I'm saying is become pro-active earlier in the year, because if you wait until October, IF you get diagnosed, which I pray you won't, your bills will be higher. I hope this helps you out.

I love you all and pray for you always. I got my nap and am feeling better than yesterday. Thank you for praying! My support team (you) is the BEST ever!

Yeah! We hit the FIVE FINGERS mark!!!

What a humbling experience. Our friends got together and planned a benefit auction for us. We are so humbled and blessed by the many friends who have jumped in to help us on this journey!

May 5th, 2014

People have been saying things and calling me names. I hardly know what to say or how to react. I am not awesome and I am not courageous. I cringe when I hear this and my gut feeling is to say, "Let me introduce you to the real Karen Weber!"

I am not awesome, but I do serve an awesome God! I am awe struck! I am in awe of Him! I am not courageous either. I wish I had more courage, but the truth is they just could have possibly named the chicken dance after me! Braaack, braack brack!

I am such a big chicken that the nurse who takes my five gallons of blood each week told Joe that they baby me!!! I get the baby needles! They also match my bandage strips to my outfit each week. How cool is that! I'm such a baby in there, I wouldn't be surprised if they offer me Hello Kitty bandages one of these days! The only reason I don't have a sticker chart is probably because they haven't thought of it.

No, I'm not courageous, I'm just like you. Except you still have beautiful hair, fingernails, eyelashes and all of your body parts. Having courage is something I definitely struggle with.

I believe a person just eats what is put on their plate. I sit there and move it all around and play in it before I ever take a bite. It's like you have to sit there until you clean it up. Like you, I don't always like what's on my plate, but there's not much I can do about it. Nobody seems to want to trade plates!

Right now one of the things I am struggling with is wearing summer clothes in public. As long as I can wear a jacket or a scarf around my neck, I don't look so much like a boy! I have a hard time going without those and with the weather warming up, I know I have to convince myself it doesn't matter. I know that no one is going to laugh at me or tease me. I guess it's vanity that makes one want to feel adequate and look normal like everyone else. But I'm not normal anymore. I know some of you are going to say that I never was normal (by the way I know who you are too) BUT I thought I was normal!!

I'm also struggling with having to wear a hat all the time. I'm ready to pitch it! I'm afraid my bald head would blind you! Again I struggle with my vanity. Sometimes I wonder if chemo is taking me so long because I just haven't learned the lesson I'm supposed to learn yet

Some tell me that I'm courageous because I'm telling my story. But I'm not! I'm telling my story because I'm afraid to walk alone! You're the ones who are brave! You walk right along beside me, not knowing anymore where I'm going than I do, and yet, you keep right on encouraging me and helping me be able to take the next step because I know you are on your knees or bowing your head praying for me again and again. It is your courage that has helped me keep going! It is your faithfulness and I think you are awesome!

May 10th, 2014

Have you ever received a gift that meant so much to you that you were speechless??? Have you ever received a gift that you didn't even know you wanted it... until you received it! I hardly know where to start to tell you about my blessing this week!!

Maybe it all started those many, many years ago when I was born on my Grandpa Kelly Miller's birthday. Grandpa was special to me and I was special to him. We shared birthdays and that made it so! Grandpa died when I was 13 years old. My main memories about him was snuggling up beside him and listening to him visiting with my parents. Or listening to him play his fiddle. He could make a fiddle talk!!!

We lived in Ohio when I grew up and Grandpa lived in West Virginia. It was always dark by the time we arrived at his house and he was always in bed. Grandma Lora always explained to us that he went to bed with the chickens!! Then she'd holler up the stairs to him and he'd come down and visit awhile before we all went to bed. As a child I always wondered where the chickens were and why he slept with them!!!

I also have a very special aunt. Aunt Bonnie is the youngest of my dad's six sisters! We also have some things in common.

Apparently when we pout; we stick our bottom lip out. Dad always threatened to step on mine if I didn't suck it back in when I was little. I've always loved my Aunt Bonnie.

There are several cartoon artist in our family. Some of us like to draw heads, dogs with a knot in their tails etc. It all started with Grandpa. If there was an envelope, a piece of paper or edge of newspaper around, you could bet Grandpa had drawn a picture on it.

Five years ago, my Aunt Bonnie took some of those pictures and made them into a quilt! Yep! You can't help but guess it.... That quilt has been gifted to me! Don't leave yet! The best is yet to come!!!

Aunt Bonnie didn't plan on making this quilt for me. I daresay she probably made it for herself or one of her daughters or granddaughters. All I know is that this was a project five years ago. I'm pretty sure it did not enter her mind at the time that she was making it for me.

Recently Aunt Bonnie had a dream in which Grandpa Kelly told her to give the quilt to ME. He said in her dream that he wanted me to have it so when I looked at it (how can I see it through my tears!) it would help me kick cancer! She went on to tell me in her letter about the day I was born and how he was called first by my parents since I was born on his birthday! She also spoke of how proud he was of me.

I was speechless when I opened this gift and read the letter. I cannot express how much it means to me! I cannot even express how much her letter means to me! A gift that anyone who knew Grandpa Kelly would have loved to have (herself included) and yet she gifted it to me. I am humbled. I love you more than words can say and I thank you from the bottom of my heart.

I pray God will bless you abundantly for your precious gift and generosity. Included with the quilt was a beautiful pendant of a turtle and a sea shell from my cousin Terry. (Aunt Bonnie's daughter) You all are the best and I can't wait to see you all!! Love, love, love you all!!! I will always cherish your gifts and dream!!! I feel like I've been given a gift from heaven!!! Thank you Grandpa Kelly! I love you so much!

May 12th, 2014

I've got my BLING on.... Big Bad Bull.... you'd better think about running!!! I plan on riding you tomorrow and I plan on winning!!!! Aww you poor Big Bad Bull!!!

May 14th, 2014

Last Thursday I was sitting in the lab room waiting with my dad I was there to get another blood test. I'm not sure how much blood I even have left. By my calculations, I could be running low! I don't like needles of any kind and I don't like bandages that rip the skin right off of you! Like many others, I feel that little room is one to dread.

Like I said, I was sitting there waiting and there was a man sitting across from me. He spoke up and said "May I ask you a question?" I of course said "yes". He asked "Do you have cancer?"

I wondered what gave him the clue; my boyish figure or lack of hair on top! Just a thought, but lack of hair does not by any means mean lack of brains!!! I told him that I used to have cancer but now I'm on preventive measures to keep it from coming back. We chatted a bit.

He asked about my journey. I found out he was just diagnosed. It was his first trip. He'd never been sick a day in his life and now he was 68 and facing the BIG C word. I found out we have the same Doctor. I also found out he was scared spitless!!!

I remember sitting in his chair. I remember it like it happened today! I remember the feelings! When the Big C word is slapped on you; your life changes forever. I remember when the Doctor told me I was stage IIIC and I asked her for how long. When would it go backwards? She told me I would always be considered a Stage IIIC. I remember how angry that made me feel. It's like being told you'll never walk again and yet you look down and you see two legs and you say "oh yes I will!!"

I watched "Mr. Man's" face and I saw the fear! I heard it in his voice. I felt it as he reached out to me! I am so thankful I had the opportunity to encourage him that day. I'm so thankful that I was ahead of him on the walk and could let him know he wouldn't walk it alone.

Some days I sit and think about how much cancer has robbed from me. Well, generally I'm standing not sitting, in front of the bathroom mirror. I look at my bald head, my chopped up body, and the circles under my eyes. I think of the hours I've spent sitting in my chair.

I look at the piles of clothes that no longer fit my boyish figure. I look at my missing eye lashes, my missing finger nails and my fading eyebrows. I look at my left arm and know I can't carry a purse on that side or lift like I used to. I can never have my blood pressure taken on that side. I look at my house that resembles a tornado going through it.

I watch Joe walk out of the house to get groceries and pay bills and so wish I wasn't too tired to ride along. I open the windows and listen to him mowing grass and wish I was out there working in the yard with him. I listen to phone calls from my kids and wish I could travel and visit them. I get a call from my grandbabies and just wish I had the strength to be with them all day.

I wish I could go in Walmart and not just go straight to the item I want, but had the strength to walk around and see what's new and visit with everyone I see that we know. I wish that, but instead I grab a cart to lean on and get the item I need and head to the door where Joe waits with the car at the entrance. I wallow in the pity party of poor me! It gets me nowhere.

In a split second these thoughts go through my head as "Mr Man" reaches out to me in that scary blood sucking lab room. I dread the journey for him. I want to yell.... RUN! RUN out that door! Run for your life!!

Instead my eyes light up and I reach back to him. I tell him how excited I am that we share the same Doctor and how wonderful she and all of the nurses are too. I tell him how he will love everyone in the chemo room. I tell him of the new medications and the new test and how he's joined a new family now, where there's love and support. We share names and promise to pray for each other. I tell him, he won't walk this journey alone. I tell him he CAN do this!!! I tell him all the wonderful things you all have been telling me!

Yes, Cancer robs you of a lot of things. It's not an easy journey by any stretch of the imagination. BUT.... I cannot count the many blessings we have had because of cancer. I was not prepared to be blessed so much. The prayers, the friends, the family, the hugs, the tears shared, the little surprise gifts, the flowers, the cards, the meals.

Strangers, friends and family, Doctors and nurses, fellow cancer patients, support teams. I am over whelmed with the care of each of you. Our church has been a support team like I've never seen before. Friends and community have not grown wearing of cheering me on and praying for me! YOUR prayers for me have amazed me!!

Yes, cancer robs you, it humbles you in a way I've never been humbled before. It's taken my confidence at times and robbed me of my dignity. But God has blessed me more than I can comprehend. He has poured out his grace and cuddles me under His wings. He has allowed me to know every step of the way HE has walked with me and HE has carried me. HE has built my confidence, my patience, my understanding and my love.

To show me He has given me more wisdom, He's even given me gray hair. Does He have a sense of humor or what!!! HE has built my support team. He has heard the prayers of my heart even when I've been so chemo brain, I couldn't pray. He's never left my side. I honor HIM! I praise HIM! I worship HIM! HE gets ALL the praise! Yes "MR Man"... Satan may have reared his ugly head and nipped at your heels but just remember... God ALWAYS wins!! Keep walking and pick up speed. Keep running to HIM! Help me pray for "MR Man". Will you? I'm still praying for you too!!!

I was so blessed to get to go to the Methodist church and speak today. It was my opportunity to bless them for blessing me with the prayer quilt they had made for me. I had my notes with me but, it seems I didn't follow them quite like I wanted to. For one thing, I wrote at the top of my notes in bold letters:

NO CRYING!!!! As I spoke and looked out at the faces that had gathered to hear me, I observed several eyes looking back at me with tears in them and some had even slipped down on their cheeks. It's hard to see your notes when that happens! I do want to share with you my thoughts! I had been thinking and praying about what I could say to encourage these souls for the generous blessing of the prayer quilt that they had made and given to me. Here are my thoughts and I tried to keep to them as best as possible:

Greetings! I am high on chemo right now since I took a treatment yesterday. Chemo affects your memory and your thinking, so I hope I don't forget what to say! (Actually I did forget somewhat and wasn't even able to read most of my notes) When I get mixed up on what I want to say, it just makes me want to pull my hair out and we don't want that for sure!

It impressed me they put my name on the quilt. I don't like being a number. I'm glad that even though God numbers us amongst HIS people, He KNOWS OUR NAME! He knows YOUR name! He knows MY name! He writes our names in His book of life but he does number the heads under our hair! (Yes, I really said it that way) That's called chemo brain! I like to try to picture what God writes by my name.

Karen Weber: (maybe He draws a little flower to acknowledge I'm a girl even though I'm flat like a boy now)

One head.... 136 hairs (that's not much) 3 eye lashes... one on the left... 2 on the right. Do you realize how off balanced that makes a person? It's difficult to put mascara on just three eyelashes! Your eyes tend to follow the eye with the most lashes!! Do you realize what your eyelashes do for you? They keep your eyes from sticking together!

The Pink Duck

If I shut my eyes, it's not because I'm falling asleep. It's because I can't get my eyes unstuck because my eyelashes have fallen out!

Karen Weber: (Little flower) One head, 125 hairs, eleven lost in the shower today. ZERO eye lashes... all gone now.... Talks too much...

I think what must have happened to me was, last summer I was really hot! Not knowing it was the estrogen from the cancer, I thought it was just the hope and change that we'd been promised and I was just hoping I would make it through the change! A modest lady by nature I was shedding clothes like a mad woman. I would often say "If I could... I think I would just shave my head!" I think I must have said it one time too many and God pointed His finger at me and said "I'll take care of that and change you in the process!"

Last summer I also asked in a prayer request, that our prayer team would pray for me that I would not be lazy! I'm not a lazy person, I'm a Martha personality. I like to "get 'er done!" But I kept feeling like I just wanted to sit down more than I needed to. I feared I was getting lazy. God obviously heard that to. I'm not sure if He got it from an e-mail or a conversation I had.

He whapped me down on the potter's wheel to remake me! All the time I'm thinking, "I can't do this, I talk too much, and I can't sit still either!" Do you know how dizzy you get when you're on the potter's wheel! It's time for a "Be still and know that I am God" time of your life! It's time for the ride of your life!

God strips you of who you are and you're more aware of who HE is! He's got one hand on the inside working out the stones and the other on the outside forming you and caressing you to make you into what HE wants.

Karen Weber: Little flower, one head, 147 hairs (growing) still no eye lashes, still talks too much, sitting better, grateful heart is growing, pride gone (pretty much) thankful, getting back on course....starting to trust ME (God) more!

When Judy Thompson called me to bring out the gift, I had no idea what she was bringing. I guessed it was maybe another box of chocolates, or a book, maybe some flowers. I never dreamed that a whole church was praying for me! I never dream of a quilt with knots tied all over it signifying prayers for ME. For ME!!!! Karen Weber!!! For little ole, bald headed ME!!! I never dreamed such a gift would reach down and touch my soul!

I felt like a card just wasn't adequate to thank each one for your prayers. I didn't want to just be quilt number 158 or whatever number of quilts you had made. I didn't want you to just know my name! I wanted to be a blessing back to you. I have felt the knots in my beautiful quilt over and over and over. I take naps under this quilt and I pray for you each. Thank you from the very bottom of my heart.

May 16th, 2014

Your have never really lived....until you have done something for someone who can never repay you!! I don't know who said that...but it is so true!

This was a good post for me to see today. I LOVE doing things for others, however today I find myself sitting in my chair again, knowing others are doing for me. I am so humbled at how our friends, family, church and community have rallied around us. My thought is a constant "How can I ever repay everyone"! I thank you from the bottom of my heart for your love and care! I can hardly wait to get back to work to pay it forward. Your care is such an inspiration and I thank God for each of you and pray for you always!!

May 22nd, 2014

The Lady in the mirror caught my eye! She looked a bit familiar to me and I gave her a second glance. I'm pretty sure she's older than me. She might even look a little like I might look like years from now! Her hair is... well I don't mean to be mean, but its short! Like really short and scraggly with a brown/gray color. I'd not be caught with my hair that short or color! Her face is void of expression as she catches me staring at her. I've caught her eye too. I wonder about her.

She's way older than me, far wiser according to her short hair. I study the laughter lines around her eyes, she's surely lived a happy life! I look closer as this lady who has fascinated me stares back at me. I see the deep ugly red scars on her body and swiftly avert my face, but my eyes are drawn back to her eyes. I realize that the tears running down her cheeks are running down mine, that her tears... are my tears! I gasp as the truth of the lady hits me! I know her far too well and I don't know her at all. Who is this lady I call me?

My husband has pictures of me in various places around our home. I look at them smiling back at me and think..."Now THAT is ME!" I'm happy, cheerful, oh so young! And yet... it's not me! I'm not the same girl! I've learned too much, traveled too far. I've been through too much! I look back at the lady in the mirror.... still watching me and I think... Is that really me??

I like to learn! I like the details! Sometimes I want to know too much! Sometimes I don't want to know some of the things I know. Sometimes I ask too many questions. "So just what are you telling me?" I asked my doctor today. I had been asking her what my survival rate was and what chances were of this "C Monster" returning again in this sink or swim world.

It was supposed to be a happy, happy day! My youngest son sat beside me in the doctor's office. It was one of those "doin' your mama proud" days! He had a job interview going on that morning and had just received good grades at law school. He was dressed in a suit and tie and looked mighty handsome. At over 6'4" he towers above me. He has his own special

Just Cleaning Up My Plate!

charisma and he's my baby boy! I love him without question (as I do all 3 of my sons!) Today he's going with his mama to support her and help her ride the bull! Mama is going to show him how it's done!

Oh happy, happy day!

I blink with my "gone with the chemo" no eyelashes eyes! I repeat the doctor's words back to her! "You're telling me with all this chemo and doing radiation, my chance of NOT getting cancer again is...60%?!!!" (Isn't 60% a failing grade?) I wanted 99% at the least 85%! I reply as my heart sinks! You're saying had I not done chemo and radiation according to the computer, I wouldn't be here in 10 years!" (I know my math! I was #2 in Math in Junior High. I graduated 40 years go and am still 39! I can handle new math! I know my numbers and how they work!)

Proud Mama's son, who hasn't said a word yet chimed in! "That's better than a fifty/fifty chance Mom!" I realize he was with me on a cruise once when I wanted to learn how to work a slot machine! We'd decided to learn together! Did I really ask to borrow 20 bucks when I lost my $20 limit of quarters! Did he really refuse me the 20 bucks because he thought I was having too much fun and might have a gambling streak? I weigh his words, knowing 50% usually means "game on" for me!

But my heart had already sunk! It had already reached the pit of my stomach and was slowly working its way back into place. Could I really go through this again if it returned? Is all of this for naught anyway!

Doctor Nevils must have read my thoughts. She reassured me and punched my confidence buttons. "These are only book numbers and you know ONLY God knows the real facts! These numbers don't have to mean anything! Live your life!" She shared amazing survivor stories with me. I mentally kicked myself because I'd even asked!! In fact... had insisted on knowing! I nod! After all, there's a bit of the gambler in my blood that chemo didn't kill. I've always like a good challenge. Although I wouldn't call this a "good" challenge. The stakes are high! But I do happen to be on the winning team. It's a win/win situation anyway you look at it.

I look back at the lady in the mirror. Yes, she's me, today that is! A little scared, frustrated, wishing for more, a bit more serious, feeling like time has flown and a whole lot wiser. I smile back at "me" and wipe the tears from my cheeks. My heart goes to the verse God gave me nine months ago when I stood before the mirror with this same lady, frustrated! Jeremiah 29V11 "I know the plans I have for you - plans to prosper you and not harm you - to give you hope and a future". Prosper... what's that? He's talking about blessings, prayer warriors, more Jesus. He's talking growth and drawing closer. He's talking... "I'm going to pour out my blessings in a way that you'll know it's the GREAT I AM!" He's talking about holding my hand all the way! He's talking about you praying for me and me praying for you!

The lady in the mirror smiles back at me. That's my girl she says! Get out there and live! Yes, it is a happy, happy day. I know in whom I have believed and am persuaded HE will keep me! My "sons" - you do your mama proud! I love you each to the moon and back! Pray for me as I pray for you!

I'm going to dance 'til the cows come home! I want to know the moves when I dance those streets of gold! Computer VS God... Who do you think wins????

May 23rd, 2014

Such a beautiful spirited friend! Thanks for visiting me in chemo today Colleen Hills!

Thank you for my gift! (I am not afraid of tomorrow for I have seen yesterday and love today!)

Counting down with my baby sister! Love her to the moon and back!

My hubby is having fun riding the mules tonight! I cannot wait to ride the mules! It's about time to stop bull riding and start mule riding!!! Such a happy, happy day having my youngest son James here to support me with my bull riding! Love you son to the moon and back!!! Thanks for going with me!!!

May 26th, 2014

Thanking you all in advance for the prayers for my last bull ride! I'll be praying for you too!!! It's what we do! Huh!!!

May 27th, 2014

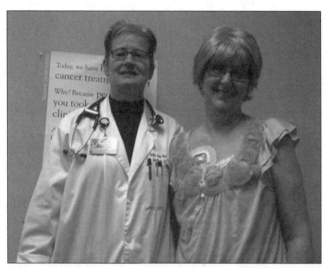

DR Nevils and me at my last chemo visit. I was gifted this blond wig. I've never been blond before. Think I can pull it off??? Well, I did... (Pull it off) after about 30 minutes.

What fun to have a pink balloon lift off at the clinic with friends and family!!! Thank you to all who attended to help me celebrate my big day!!! We did it!!! We conquered the bull and lifted our hands to the sky, praising God!!

I was more than excited! Today... that BIG BAD BULL would be no match for me! He was snorting and pawing the ground! Still, I hopped on his back and hung on for the ride. My last ride! I was more than anxious! I was more than ready! A feeling I'd not had with any of the previous rides thundered through my veins! All I could think was "get 'er done and over with"!

In my mind, I was too excited to be afraid! Too excited to even consider this would still be a rough ride! I was too excited for anything but to have this last ride over with! BIG BAD BULL was flexing his muscles causing mine to jerk and I was hanging on for dear life when I happened to see you!

"You" were new in the chemo room. I hadn't seen you before. You still had a full head of beautiful hair! Your eyelashes were still intact. I noticed you because our mutual friend (Your new friend and my friend for the past nine months) was visiting with you.

I watched our friend walk over and get the box of hats and began to show you the many different ones and explain ideas to you. I watched you look over the hats and feel them. I watched the look on your face. I closed my eyes and I began to pray for you! Tears came to my eyes and I silently cried for you!

Our nurse navigator is such an awesome lady. She's going to be one of your best friends for the next while. I watch you as you listen intently to her and somehow... I know your thoughts.

You can't even comprehend what she's saying. You know "what" she's saying, but it's like it's happening to another person. How can it be you she's speaking of? You haven't even adjusted to the "C" word yet. You're learning about hats, and scarves and wigs and you can't even take it in yet that your beautiful thick hair will be gone in maybe a week or two! You can't comprehend YOU being bald! It doesn't seem possible.

Tears well up in my eyes again as I think of all you are going to face. My hand glides over my own bald head and my heart cries for what you don't even know yet. I cling tighter to the bull I am riding and the tears slip down my checks! I don't want you to see me, for I am in pain for the journey for you. You are a stranger to me, and yet I share your pain.

I pray you are strong. I pray you get good reports and that you have a strong support team. I pray you have faith. I pray you beat this monster!

My ride is over! I slide over the side of the heavy breathing bull. My legs, weak from the thunderous ride! It's my day to celebrate and the nurses bring the singing bear and clap and sing for me. We celebrate my last bull ride! I have been looking forward to this day for nine long months. I didn't expect to cry! All of the nurses are clapping and dancing for this happy day for me! Every one of them are beautiful and they touch my heart. They have helped me ride this bull for sixteen thunderous rounds! Smiles puff our cheeks and tears of joy fill our eyes! We group hug!

Yet...my thoughts return to you... beginning your journey as I've just finished my last ride. You notice me and my celebration! The whole room celebrates with me! I want more than ever for my last ride and celebration to give you courage! I want you to know you can do this! You can ride the BIG BAD Bull and win! I hate cancer! I hate what you are going to go through. I may have walked (staggered is more like it) out of the chemo room today, but I left a chunk of my heart right there with those still riding the bulls.

I pray for you sister that you along with the others still in treatment will have good days and good outcomes! I can't wait to see you at the SURVIVORS picnic next year! May God Bless your journey!! I'm going to be praying for you!

YEAH!!!!!! I whooped that bull!
The Last Bull Ride

Chapter 10

Normal Isn't Normal Any More

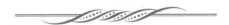

June 3rd, 2014

It's the little things that make a gal happy! I went to the Bond Clinic today. I did NOT get on the scales!!! I did NOT get chemo!! I started painting our closet today. Yep, used both arms!!! Up, down.... up... down! I got a good therapy report!!! I received two cards in the mail! We heard from two of our sons today! BLT's and corn on the cob for supper! Enjoyed the smell of green grass as hubby mowed the lawn. First Tuesday in forever that I haven't had to give blood! Yep, this gal is happy, happy, happy! I hope you are too! What makes you happy???

June 8th, 2014

We had our first free weekend where I could go out of town. Joe took me to Branson! What fun. I had lots of naps! But hey, when I was awake I had fun! So glad I'm married to a patient man!

June 10th, 2014

Feeling me some love!!! My first doctor's appointment since my last chemo! Got a good report and especially loved hearing DR Nevils say... "You are recovering from chemo!" It was like music to my ears. Hillary Thomas made me a cherry pie and delivered it today! Yes, I'm feeling loved!

June 11th, 2014

I'm going to get a lot done today, but first... I'm taking a nap!

June 16th, 2014

I am still praying for YOU!

June 18th, 2014

It's been three weeks since my last bull ride! I've been trying to "get my life back" you might say. It's not as easy as it may sound. My hair managed to fall out (a lot) again and my eyebrows are completely gone for the first time. The pain in my arms and legs has frustrated me along with the numbness in my feet and hands. These are all part of the side effects. Just one more therapy session on Thursday. I have another PET scan this week (Here Kitty, Kitty) to find out if everything is as it should be results wise since the chemo. I also find out just when radiation starts.

Today I met DR Graham and she told me I will have six and 1/2 weeks of radiation (five days a week). Previously I had been told 4 - 7 weeks. I was hoping for the four weeks. This means my treatments will continue into August!! Which means.... 12 months of my life, I will have been dealing with this! UGH!

I am thankful though that you have made this journey with me and have not grown weary of praying for me. DR Graham also clarified the numbers rolling around in my head. After I have completed radiation, I will have a 10% chance of the cancer returning in the affected area. That's pretty good and I'm happy with those numbers. However the 40% that's been aggravating me is for any other area.

I guess I need to be thinking of body parts to get rid of to lower that number! Nah, think I'll hang onto what I have left and take my chances. After all I would look funny getting rid of my bones and a person just can't enjoy life being paranoid. Hang with me a bit longer and pray that my PET scan results will show miracle results and that I will make it through the radiation without side effects. I would also ask you to pray that this numbness and pain goes away fast! After learning today how long this chemo can stay in my body... well... let's just say, side effects, please go away! I will continue to pray for you as well. Keep me posted on how you're doing!!! Hugs!

June 19th, 2014

We lost Lynn to ovarian cancer 12 years ago. Today would have been her birthday! I miss her so much! We celebrate her birthday each year with chocolate cake and drink milk and have a balloon lift off. Lynn always said she wanted to eat a whole chocolate cake and drink a gallon of milk. Miss you big sister!!!

NOT excited about my PET scan tomorrow but praying for good results!!! It seems to me this has gone on long enough!

June 20th, 2014

Leaving for my PET scan. WHERE is that cat??? Here Kitty, Kitty!

WOW! That was exhausting! Got my PET scan done and my markers for my radiation done all in the same setting, lying on a hard table with a cramp in my back. PLEASE don't move!! You're doing great.... you're a real trooper!!! No... You can't move your legs, no you can't bring yours arms down. I felt like I was hanging from the monkey bars, sideways. I knew if I lost my grip, I'd never get it back.

Now we're in the hurry up and wait phase. Expecting radiation to likely start on Wednesday. I feel like a coloring book as I have magic marker lines drawn all over me and stickers put on me in different spots. I haven't looked yet to see if they are Dora or Hello Kitty but I imagine they will be Hello Kitty since it was a PET scan! Hello!!

Before the scan I had to "sit still" for 40 minutes. Like I haven't had enough practice for that this past 10 months!!! They give you warm blankets and turn the lights out! There is nothing to do except pray. Which I did for you; until I fell asleep and they came and woke me up. I was in such pain from the cramp in my back for the actual scan and the radiation scan that I decided if I didn't want them to see me cry; I'd better start praying again!

I prayed again for little Abby Taylor who is having a double brain surgery this morning (what right did I have to feel like crying for myself!!) and then covered several other states of friends and family. Praying helped me get through it without embarrassing myself with tears.

The test itself didn't hurt of course; it was the stupid cramp in my back and not being able to move! Anyway, all is done! YOU are prayed for and I'm outta there until next week!!! Yeah!!! Thank you for your prayers!!!! I love you 'uns!!! (Yep... that's a word!)

June 21st, 2014

It amazes me that I have such amazing friends, family and strangers praying for me!! I love, love, love you!! Thank you so much for traveling this journey with me! For the constant encouragement! You will never know how much you really mean to me!!! It's my joy to pray for you as well!!! God is good.... all the time!

June 24th, 2014

PET scan results today. Radiation starts tomorrow. Almost there! Should be done with this mid-August!!! I feel like my summer is being thrown down the drain! Last year I had Thing One and Thing Two with me several days each week. They have not played in our yard once this summer. No swinging on the swing set.... no playing in the sandbox.... no time in the play house... no tea parties on the deck... no riding the bikes... no chalk writing on the concrete....no swimming or running through the sprinkler. Cancer Sucks!

June 24th, 2014

Having me a little celebration! I'm drinking Melaleuca's Gourmet Hot cocoa! It is so good that I'm about ready to lick the mug! I could get carried away; I am so excited!! I went in to get my port flushed today and for the reading of the PET scan! (NOT to be confused with the reading of the WILL!) My last PET scan was October 23, 2013. This was a comparison of the two scans! (June 24, 2014)

I'm not sure what Restaging of stage III breast cancer means as I was told I would always be considered a Stage IIIC. There's also a bunch of other big words I don't understand on the report. But I do understand most of it and I do for sure understand the bottom line. FINDINGS: No evidence of recurrent breast or chest wall mass. No evidence of axillary or sub-pectoral lymphadenopathy. (Even spell check doesn't know some of these words!) Right subclavian venous access device is in appropriate position. (That would be my port!) No evidence of mediastinal or hilar lymphadenopathy. The heart and great vessels are within normal range. The lungs are clear! There are no abdominal or pelvic masses. No adnexal masses are identified. There are no abnormal foci of metabolic activity! BOTTOM LINE: NO evidence of RESIDUAL or RECCURRENT neoplasm! Now you read that and tell me if we should shout or sing!!!

I was looking at it trying to take it all in and my doctor said.... "THIS is GOOD news Karen! This is what we want!!" I was so stunned to get such a good report; I guess she thought I wasn't responding quickly enough! It really is a good thing when you see your doctor excited!!!

I want to thank each of you for praying for me and not growing weary! It's been a long hard haul and you've stayed by my side. I know I could not do it without your prayers. I'm sure you have no idea how much you each have encouraged me on this journey. Knowing you were there cheering me on and praying consistently for me has helped me beyond words.

This week I have felt so good and have managed to get some house cleaning and organizing done. Something that drives me up a tree when it's undone. I've certainly learned that it will wait for you to get to it! Some of it is still waiting for me. That's ok.... one step at a time! Tomorrow I start the next step of my journey. At 11:15 a.m. I start my 6 1/2 weeks (5 days a week) of radiation.

I'm feeling so good right now. I dread the almost 40 mile trip every day and the feeling of being tired again but I know "This too shall pass!" At least there shouldn't be a lot of needles involved in this stretch of the journey! Hopefully NO bull rides! Since I've already licked the bottom of my hot cocoa mug; I'm going to head to bed. Sleep well tonight my friend! I'm going to say a special prayer for you!

June 25th, 2014

Here we go counting down backwards 34 - 1 First treatment #34. My nurse navigator and friend Carol Walters tells me this is just a pony ride compared to the bull ride! We'll see if I drag my feet! Let's get this done and over with!!! Come on!!!

Chapter 11

Facing the Monster

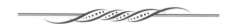

July 7th, 2014

Eight down... twenty-seven to go! I have to brag on my radiation team! They are quick and to the point! I'm only in there about 30 minutes it seems. Just about the time I think I can finally lay still and take a nap; they come in and say "Mrs. Weber... you can put your arms down now." I never seem to know if they are waking me up or if I didn't have time to fall asleep. I sure do appreciate the gospel music they turn on for me. The time is short in there and I suppose that big ole ugly machine circling me is doing its job.

One week into it and I'm feeling fine. I can drive myself coming and going! That means I can also take a side trip and make stops if I want! Wahoo! Independence is back. I have been warned that the longer that I take the treatments; I will start being tired again. For right now; I'm kickin' up my heels.

I'm very frustrated with the left over side effects of the chemo. My hands and feet are so numb they are driving me up a tree. I still can't wear my rings because of the swelling! This feeling is supposed to go away in time, but to me, it feels like it's getting worse! My energy seems to be coming back a little at a time for now and I'm enjoying catching up on the house and even "got" to pull some weeds Saturday. Never thought I'd ever say that!! I even made strawberry freezer jam tonight!

I'm STILL bald and it troubles me greatly. Joe says I can't put towels over the mirrors in the house until it grows back. He totally vetoed the idea when I suggested it. Having no eyelashes and having to draw eyebrows on every day is frustrating. It is not pretty!! You know it's the little things that count! I'll be so glad when my fingernails start to grow and I can scratch again! HAHAHA!!! Those 'ole Missouri chiggers are about to drive me nuts! Just kidding but they are bad this year! If you've got 'em... just put a dab of clear nail polish on them and it will smother them out. If you don't have them; you probably aren't in Missouri!!! It's past my bedtime. Night 'yall... I'm outta here!

July 8th, 2014

I did it!!! I entered my short story in a writers contest! "The Stranger in the Mirror" by Karen Weber. The winner will be announced on Tuesday one week from today!! I want to win... I want to win... I want to win! If I win... I'll get to publish my book earlier instead of later!!! Thank you for encouraging me to write!!! After the contest ends, I will post my story. Years ago, our radio station held a contest for writing about Ground Hog's Day. The winner won 25 pounds of "ground hog". I won the contest and won 25 pounds of sausage! The current contest will include writers from around the world! Nine treatments down with twenty-six to go!!

July 12th, 2014

Don't be alarmed if you see Joe around town. He and I am in a race to see who can grow hair the fastest. He's not shaving! So far he's ahead of me!

July 15th, 2014

Oh! I didn't want to look at the list of winners in the short writing contest, so I just looked with one eye! No, my name wasn't on the list of the top three. How disappointing! However, I still did something on my bucket list! I entered a writing contest! I did it! I did it! I did it!

If you would like to read the winning entries, you can go to Xulon Press (dot com) and read them. Congratulations to the top winners! I think everyone who entered is a winner. We got out of our comfort boxes and competed with writers around the world!

Disappointed? Yep! Down? Nope! Competitive? I compete with myself all the time! Looks like I'm going to kick it up a notch. I'd better get on that! Thanks for cheering me on anyway! I love you all and still pray for you!!!

The story I entered in the contest!

The Stranger in the Mirror

By Karen Miller Weber

I stared at the lady in the mirror looking at me. We have nothing in common. I am a vibrant, dark-eyed beauty even in my fifties. I have long flowing beautiful auburn hair. My eyelashes almost touch my dark rimmed glasses. Guessing, I would say I weigh about twenty pounds more than the lady staring back at me. I am full of energy and am always ready to kick up my heels.

It's funny, even though the lady staring back at me is a stranger to me, I know her every thought... her every pain! I study her closely. She is bald! Well almost bald. What she has stands straight up on her head. It's scraggly and I see more head than hair. It looks like it might be easy to count the hairs on her head. She has no eyebrows or eyelashes. She has dark circles under her eyes and she looks tired.

I look closer. She has no breast. She's as flat as a young boy. I run my hands down over my own body and am reminded that I have no breast either. I too am flat. Flat as a lumpy pancake! I run my hands over my head. My head with the long flowing hair! Only there is no hair! Just a few sprigs standing straight up.

I look at the lady in the mirror. Our eyes meet. Tears are flowing down her cheeks and I realize those same tears are flowing down my own cheeks. How can that stranger in the mirror be me!! How can I not recognize myself? Tears flow down faster and faster and I cannot control them.

I turn from the lady in the mirror and refuse to accept that she is me. Still, I am drawn to her. She calls me like a long lost friend. I cannot refuse the hold she has over me. It cannot be!!! I cry until I don't even recognize the sounds coming from my throat. I don't recognize the sounds coming from my heart. But I feel the pain. Heart rendering pain that is tearing me apart. "Lord! Help me!" I cry out as I drop to the floor and sob.

I pull myself together as I realize I am going down a slippery slope. I cannot afford to go there. I do not want to go there. Grabbing a clean washrag, I scrub my face as hard as I can wiping away the tears, trying to wipe even me away. Anger runs through my hurt and I recognize that my own body has betrayed me. It has allowed cancer to grow in me. How can that be? Not me! Happy, energetic, life loving me! This happens to strangers. How did it touch me? How did it sneak up on me!

I grab my toothbrush and start brushing my teeth. As I grit them it's a wonder I am not brushing the enamel off as my hurt and anger flows through me. Through clenched teeth I cried out... "This is NOT the plans I had!" Immediately God spoke to me in His calm, quiet voice and said, "I know the plans I have for you, plans to prosper you and not to harm you, plans to give you a hope and a future." (Jeremiah 29:11)

> My tears slowed and a peace came over me. Immediately I knew I was on this journey for a reason and I was not going to die. For what reason... I did not know. I don't know that I'll ever know. But God had just promised me HE was going on this journey with me. He would not leave my side. I heard it! I felt it! I knew it!
>
> Though I did not look it, I walked out of the bathroom more like my original self. Happy that God had spoken to me during the storm. He'd picked me up. He'd secured my grip on him. No matter what tomorrow brings, He has His finger on my life. I can count on it. I passed another mirror as I walked through to my recliner where I would spend the next several months. I saw my reflection, bald, no eyebrows, no eyelashes, my breast are gone. I looked and smiled...I am a stranger in this land and I am the apple of God's eye!
>
> You can read the winning entries at Xulon Press (dot com)

I'm not sure who suggested me but I thank them from the bottom of my heart! Tomorrow I get to sit in on a meeting for the new "Delbert Cancer Center" coming soon to Rolla! Five of us were chosen! Going to make some new friends and get to express our opinions, ideas and concerns! Oh!!!! I'm excited!!! Do you have any ideas you'd like brought to the table???

July 19th, 2014

Half way point! 17 down - 17 to go!!!

July 20th, 2014

WOW! I do believe the person who took over my chair this past year, has slipped in and has taken over my bed! Two hours nap yesterday afternoon and then 10 1/2 hours sleep last night!!! Who is this lady and is she going to be tasting my porridge next???

July 21st, 2014

Today was the first day in "forever" that we got to watch Thing One and Thing Two at our house! What fun we had. Loved watching Thing Two on the sea saw swing just a singing.... "My heart and my Loooorrrd. My heart and my Looorrd!!!" She was making up words as she was swinging and singing. "I love Tigers... but I want to leave them at the zoooooo..... Just me and my Loooorrrd!!!"

Thing One to me.... "Nana... I just cannot stop loving you!!!!" (Well I hope not! I'll love my girls forever!!!!!)

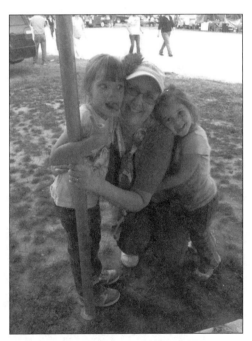

One big ball of love here!! Thing One and Two here with Nana

July 22nd, 2014

We had such fun today! Thing One, Thing Two, Papa Joe and me. We are cramming all we can into this short week! The girls are as happy to be here as we are to have them! Today Thing One told me... "The happiest days of my life are when I'm at Nana's house!"

After swimming and playing in the sandbox and eating peanut butter "sammages" and a bubble bath, the girls decided to play "dress up" again in Nana's clothes. Thing One has always favored one of my night gowns (which she wants me to give to her when she grows up). They both put on my night gowns, climbed up on the big bed and asked me to lay between them. Both snuggled up and within five minutes were sound asleep! Since both insisted they lay on one of my arms each, I was stuck and couldn't get up. It was the best stuck ever so I just laid there with them and let them sleep, absorbing their fresh clean scent. How I love those girls!!

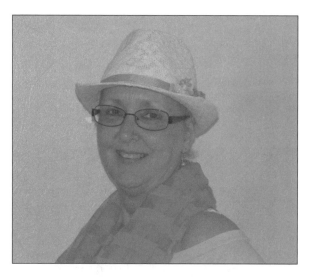

Finally updated my profile on my personal page. No hair here! But it's coming in AND these aren't fake eyebrows!!! Yeah!! They are coming back!!! Whoo hooo!! Also my eyelashes are starting to come back!! Cartwheel time!!!

July 24th, 2014

When you take radiation; the area in which you take treatments is drawn on with paint markers and you have stickers for markers. You look like a "connect the dot" coloring book. Thing One saw a part of one of the markers on my side and grabbed my shirt up and said "Oh Nana!! Did you get a tattoo!!!" Stunning art work, I must admit!! But no dear; I'm too afraid of needles to get a tattoo!
    21 down.... 13 to go!

July 27th, 2014

I am so frustrated with some of the side effects of chemo. The numbness in my hands and feet is about to make me climb the walls. I know some of you out there have had the same symptoms. What have you done about it??? Just 12 more radiation treatments to go!!! I'll be so glad when this is over with! Tired of being tired!
    My SURVIVORS "Thank you for supporting and encouraging me" party is scheduled for the last SATURDAY in October. We'll have BBQ and a balloon lift off. We will also have the quilt drawing (that Loretta Phelps made for me) at that time!! There will be mule rides and lots of music!!

July 28th, 2014

23 down... 11 to go!!

July 29th, 2014

You all are such an encouragement to me!!! I know as I get better and better that I am spending less time on the Internet. Joe mentioned today that he's noticed that I keep telling him to not drop me off at the door when we stop someplace, because I want to walk. Yes, my strength is returning. When I go to radiation, I always park at the end of the parking lot so I can get me a little walk in. Only 10 more treatments to go!!

What do you pray when you pray? Last winter a friend of mine sent me an e-mail about how she had been praying for me! Her words have rung over and over in my mind. She mentioned in Matthew 6 verse 9 where Jesus said... "This, then, is how you should pray: "Our Father in heaven, hallowed be your name, your kingdom come, your will be done, on earth as it is in heaven."

What she mentioned in her note to me was that in heaven there will be no sickness or disease! She was praying my health would be on earth as it would be in heaven! NO sickness or disease! What a gift to me her prayer is! I am very thankful for her prayer! I wonder, what if we prayed for our relationships, our families, our kids, our hearts, our thoughts, our attitudes, etc. to be on earth like they will be in heaven! Pam Feeler you have blessed me tremendously! Thank you for your prayer! Countdown is on. I'm feeling fine! I'm praying specifically for each of YOU!

July 30th, 2014

SINGLE Digits!! 25 down.... 9 to go!!! Radiation burns are like "yee-owwe"! I've been a little dizzy, so I had to have an extra little chat with the DR today. I'm having to add more B's to my diet for the chemo side effects. It's frustrating to have numb hands.

Today I bought a bottled water (I still have to drink five a day) and I couldn't open it again. The clerk had to open it for me. Talk about feeling silly!!! I'm still tired and had to have an hour and a half nap after my radiation this morning. However after lunch, I kicked up my heels a bit. I'm slowly getting there. I see the light at the end of the tunnel!! Whooo Hoooo......

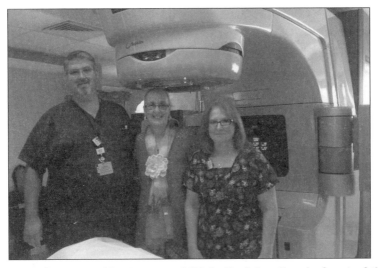

My radiation team Kent, me and Michelle (standing in front of the "monster"!!)

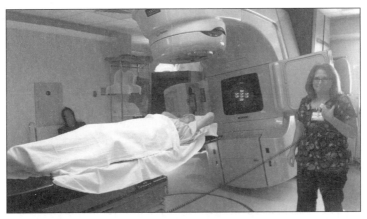

That's me getting ready for the "monster" to do its job. Nurse Michelle checks last minute markings.

CHAPTER 12

Slaying the Dragon

August 4th, 2014

Oh man!!! I am not on the 34 treatment program after all. I'm on the 36 treatment program. That means I have EIGHT more treatments to go instead of six! That is not what I wanted to hear this morning! Oh well.... what's two more treatments after 16 chemo and 28 radiation treatments! Oh nap time; here I come! I sure am "Tard"!

August 8th, 2014

There's not a thought in my head! Funny huh!!!

August 9th, 2014

Well.... I knew it couldn't last.... my brain is spinning!!
    The ole monster has turned into a dragon! They have pulled his face down and he has blown fire at me all week. Now I have gel packs on to help with the burns and swelling. A+ visit with my surgeon yesterday for follow-up. I don't have to see him again until next year unless I get my port out this year! Just four more trips to visit with "The Dragon"! Whooopeeee! My heart aches for those I've learned about who are just starting

this journey. I know you can do it! But I know it's a difficult path to climb. Remember, I'll be praying for you!!!

August 11th, 2014

Had my time with the "Dragon" today. Just three more to go!!!!

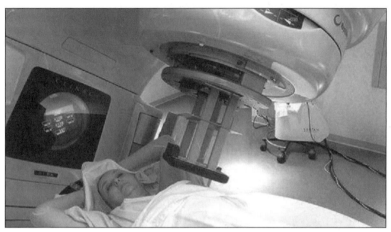

Me and "The Dragon"!

August 12th, 2014

Have you ever done some dumb thing and hoped nobody saw it! My Joe likes to keep his ducks in a row. I'm prone to scatter them and get a kick out of it as I do. I do however like nice rows of things! Like rows and rows of crops! I think they are beautiful. I also like rows of beautiful colored things. Like stacks and rows of different bright colored towels. (Red...green....orange...yellow...)

One thing I do not like is a long row of cars; with myself way back in the line. I've got that gene that says if it's in front of me I need to pass it! Yesterday while driving through town I wondered why there was about a ten car lineup in front of me and why it was creeping so! I knew I couldn't pass all ten of them at once or any for that matter as it was a no passing zone, but I did wonder why we were creeping, so I slipped over towards the yellow line so I could read the sign of the vehicle way up in front of us. Ah wet paint! Now the two tires on the driver side of my vehicle are yellow!!!!! Can't hide that!!! Oh well, at least the yellow streak isn't up my back!

Just TWO more trips to visit the DRAGON and I'll be done!!! Today, I am enjoying listening to the young man working in the yard. He whistles as he works!!!

August 13th, 2014

I am going to slay the dragon tomorrow!!! It's my very last treatment! Oh joy! Joy! Joy!!!!! I am burnt... I itch.... and I am tired, but that is nothing compared to my excitement!! You all have stayed the journey with me! You amaze me!!! I love you and I thank you! I am still praying for each of you!

August 14th, 2014

I'm on my way to slay the dragon!!! We spar off, eyeball to eyeball at 9 a.m. He may spray his fire out at me today but I'll be the winner and it will be his last time!!! I'm going to walk out of there with my head high and a new spring to my step! BOING....BOING....

I DID IT!!!! I DID IT! I DID IT!!! I slayed the Dragon and left him belly side up; laying on the floor!!! Oh what a happy day!! I did not expect to be emotional at this last treatment!!! I expected instead to be able to turn a cartwheel since I'd been told I could turn one after radiation (though I've never been able to turn one before).

I learned something I didn't know about the treatment room today. The door to the room is probably over a foot thick!!! It slides in the wall and I'd never noticed it before! It's a big scary door and seals you in the room all by yourself. I would have freaked out if I'd seen it before. I am more than happy to leave that ole Dragon in there with the door shut.

I am here to tell you... if you live in this area you will get superior treatment from the Rolla team! I am in awe of every one of them. I can hardly believe this day is finally here!!! So happy! Thank you each for praying for me through sixteen chemo treatments, two surgeries, pet scans, cat scans, thirty six radiation treatments and hard telling how many blood draws!!!! Hugs everyone!!!!

August 16th, 2014

Seriously.... when something is done; you expect it to be done! I did not expect tears for my last treatment. I expected to walk out cheering! Which I did! However I did have tears of joy, tears of relief and of accomplishment! Kent told me, I am now part of the family and I would be returning for checkups for years and years. Ok... I get that.

Regular checkups, just like at the dentist. Prevention is good medication. I hope you are keeping up with your checkups too. What I don't get is having to take it easy. I feel like I've done my time!

Yesterday to celebrate, Joe and I went to the state fair. It was fun to walk around and see all of the vendors and their exhibits. Three hours of walking and the neuropathy is like YIKES!

I was glad to return home and get to bed. Not being able to sleep for the pain, I was up, soaking my feet and waiting for the pain to go down. I didn't get to bed until almost 3 a.m. I was up early enough the next day BUT, back to bed for most of the day. What time I'm up I'm back in my chair. UGH... so ready to be back to normal! What IS normal now? I'd like to hear from some of you, telling me how you got back to normal and how long it took!

August 24th, 2014

Today was checkup day with my chemo DR. I got a good report but was disappointed that I DO have to leave my port in for another YEAR! This is one accessory that I don't enjoy wearing so I was hoping DR would say... "Hey! Let's just get that thing out of there!" She did not give me those coveted words. The reason, I was given that I need to keep it in, is because of possible relapse. I totally trust my DR and her judgment of her and her six DR team. So... I will leave it in but I'm telling you... I'm NOT going to forget my cream that numbs the area, the next time I go for a port flush!

Thank you Joe for holding my hand and Thank you Nurse Hillary Bleckman for not hurting when you "poked" me! I feel like I'm a big girl now! I am still dealing with radiation burns from the Fire Breathing Dragon. These are not pretty so I'm still on antibiotics and gel packs. I am however getting stronger every day. Most of my naps are short and sweet and I awake refreshed and ready to kick up my heels again.

I don't expect to sit on the sidelines for long. There's a lot of new folks being diagnosed with cancer and I'm asking you each to pray for them. I have two friends starting chemo tomorrow!!! Also pray that mine will not return and that this ole port will just be a precaution and nothing more. I do love praying for YOU!

August 25th, 2014

I'm pretty sure it's the Vanilla Coffee Frappe from Break Time that's keeping my brown eyes wide awake tonight. I don't think the four pieces of toast with the home made grape freezer jam have anything to do with it! (Did I really just eat four?)

I'm wide awake and it's bedtime. I'm not one that can lie in bed. Well I can, in the mornings. There's something about Mr. Sun peeping through the windows that can make a soul just want to lie there and snuggle one more shuteye out of an imaginary feather bed. But not tonight... It's Mr. Moon who beckons me out of my snuggle and onto my chair. That's usually a sign either my mind is spinning or I've had too much caffeine. It's a bit of both tonight.

I was thinking of this roller coaster of a ride I've been on this past year. I've never liked roller coasters and the truth is... I've only ever been on one. "Fire in the Hole" took me down at Silver Dollar City more than... well let's just say a LONG time ago. It probably isn't wise to take your first roller coaster ride on a ride that goes through the dark with train whistles screaming all around you. My relief of the trains not colliding on the rails that hot summer day had me swearing off of roller coasters forever.

That is... until last September, when I hopped on this "All aboard for the Bond Clinic, step this way" roller coaster ride. Truth is, the ride is just about done. We were chug, chug chugging to the finish line, I had one leg out of the buckled in seat and was dragging my foot, about to hop out when I got the call.

Now different things can set a person off on a tangent or whatever you want to call it. It was there, at that point that I found out the ride wasn't quite over. I was in for another bit of a different kind of dip! I think over the past few months, I may have told more than I intended to tell on my journey, but it is my journey and this is just one more step of it.

Generally I blame the chatter box on the chemo, but since that is over, I'll blame it on the Vanilla Coffee Frappe from Break Time, this time. I'm sure it's never just me talking, as I'm generally pretty quiet (I think....). No, I don't always think, but that's a different story.

The call was a part of my journey and I was stunned as I listened to the words on the other end of the line. In fact, neither chemo nor caffeine came to my rescue. I listened in silence to the silence on the other end of the line, until the voice spoke up and said... "Did I lose you?"

The lady on the other end had just expressed to me that bald people freak her out and since we were going to be taking a class together in the near future, she wanted to meet with me prior to the class to.... help her not be freaked out or something like that! I'm not entirely sure what she said for sure because I freaked out when she said bald heads freaked her out. What my mind heard, was... "MY bald head was going to freak her out and she needed to "test drive" the experience to see if she'd be able to take the class with me!" (After all, since I am the leader of the class, it would be hard to just ignore me)

The roller coaster gave a surprise jerk and I tucked my leg back in and held on tight! I'm not going to ask you what you would have said, because I'm pretty sure your answers would be all over the page and I'm too much of a lady to say what went through my head. I did repent!!! So why am I telling you? I don't know. I guess I'm just sharing a part of the journey that I didn't expect to happen and I can see the funny side of it now.

I've never been told I might freak somebody out before! Have you? I really was minding my own business when the phone rang that day! I hate being snuck up on my blind side. Don't you? Has anything ever come out of your mouth that you wished you'd not said? Oh my... it sure has mine, more than once. Lord have mercy on me!

What I wanted to say, was... I'll tell you what freaks me out! Leaning your head over the tub and watching your hair fall out in gobs. Yes, that freaks me out! Having a Doctor explain to you that he's going to cut part of your body off so you can live, freaks me out. Having chemo thundering through your veins freaks me out. Having a fire breathing radiation dragon breathe out fire on me, freaks me out. Not having eye lashes freaks me out! Having food taste like chemo freaks me out! That big door on the radiation room freaks me out!!! Needles freak me out! Getting a call from another friend who has just been diagnosed really freaks me out!

I was grateful my eyelashes had grown enough to catch the tears that gathered on them. I could grab them before they smeared my cheeks. Something held my tongue and I said nothing. At least I don't think I said anything.

It's taken me a few days but I realized there are different things that freak all of us out. You would laugh if you knew some of the things that freak me out! I'm not going to tell you as too many of my friends are pranksters! They might jump on the payback plan instead of the pay it forward plan.

As far as I know, I haven't lost a single friend from being bald. In fact, I've gained so many more! I've got another new group of friends and we're all bald! Yeah, we've got a bit of fuzz up there and it's as soft as a new puppy, but compared to what we were; we still feel bald. But who cares? Certainly not me!

I'm sitting here looking at all of these pictures of so many of you who have had your smiling picture taken with me and just noticed... You all have hair! You each have beautiful, never had a bad hair day in your life hair.... and I don't. I guess I've got so comfortable with being bald that I've forgotten that it might startle someone else.

I have to laugh at last summer, when my hair was so long and healthy at how many times I said... "I'm so hot, if I could I would just shave my head!" I'm NOT saying that again! Or how about this one? "That just makes me want to pull my hair out!" DON'T say it!!!

Maybe we all need to be a little more careful with what we say and how it affects others. I know I do! My leg is back out and my toe is dragging the ground trying to pull this ride to a stop. Bet I'm going to have to go shoe shopping for another pair of shoes from dragging it so much. I hope there's a pair in every color! Yes! I'd like that!!! Yes! I would!!!!

Chapter 13

Coming Full Circle Makes Me Dizzy!

September 1st, 2014

Not long ago, I was riding with a friend to the funeral of another friend of ours. We had both lost a mutual friend to cancer. It didn't even seem like a fair race for our friend Ronnie. Not many weeks earlier he had been diagnosed with three different cancers and had just had his first chemo treatment. He had lost his battle before he'd hardly had a chance to fight.

    We both felt guilty that we were still alive. I felt guilty because I had made it through the treatments and was/am doing well. My friend told me she felt guilty because she'd had cancer and hadn't had to go through what I had gone through this past year. I didn't know what to say when she expressed these feelings to me. But I do understand how she felt.

    My heart plummets to my stomach every time I hear of someone else being diagnosed. It seems like the cancer monster is more popular than the stomach flu. What's with that? Where is it coming from? Why can't we get a handle on it? I don't know the answers but I do know there are a lot of people out there needing lots of prayers. We've got to get on our knees!

September 17th, 2014

My bed isn't even made!!! Which is unusual as that's generally the first thing I do each morning. I like to climb into a neat made bed each night and I like to look in our bed room and see a nice made bed during the day with the umpteen pillows (three of which are pillows with pictures of our three sons on them). There's something soothing about having your bed made for the day. I feel like I'm up and raring to go, when my bed is made. It's like it's one of those steps that gets your day started right.

Today... it's not made, because I laid in it a little longer, listening to the rain pitter patter on our red tin roof. I lay there listening and relaxing and all of a sudden I noticed my fingers were itching to get to my keyboard to talk with you! I might warn you; my nose might be shiny and my short, short, real short hair... might appear oily! Why? Because God has been pouring (I might say dumping) out the oil of blessing on me! He has amazed me again and I am THANKFUL!

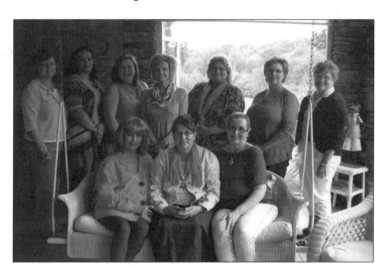

I'm not going to say how the ladies were chosen to sit around the lunch table with me yesterday, because there were many others who could have sat around that table for various reasons. (Including YOU) So many of you have carried me this past year! So many of you have lifted up my husband Joe.

As I looked around the table I knew it could have been men sitting there instead of these ladies. Men who prayed for us, brought firewood or thawed our frozen water pipes. Men who texted Joe morning and evenings to ask about us, see if there was a need or simply to say again..."I'm praying for you both today!"

I looked around the table at these ladies who had dropped their own schedules for the afternoon and came to celebrate my life, my health... our God! Bonnie sat to the right of me. I had never met Bonnie before (in person) until yesterday! She surprised me and came up all the way from Mississippi to meet me! Oh how I love surprises! Especially this kind! Bonnie was a friend of a friend! We met through cards, and phone calls and flowers. Bonnie took it upon herself to pray for me (a stranger to her) this year. I don't know what made her do that, but I am thankful for Bonnie and thankful that Sarah was so willing to share one of her best friends with me!!! Bonnie is a heart friend as beautiful as her big heart is and I loved her instantly!!!

Next to Bonnie, sat Cathy! Cathy is our pastor's wife and a mother in Israel lady. Cathy has been such a blessing in my life. It began many years ago before my bull riding days! Cathy and Pastor Dave were there for each of my surgeries, my pet scan. When I was sick and Joe needed to run for medicine, Cathy would run over and sit with me. Every time I was fearful of the next step, they were there, praying for and encouraging me! I am so thankful for Cathy! I love you more than cupcakes too Cathy!!! Beside Cathy, sat Loretta.

Loretta and I go back years. We've shared a lot of laughter and tears. We have cried 'til the snot flowed and laughed 'til we snorted!! We've been in party plan together and traveled together. I think Loretta took it personal when I was diagnosed and she hasn't left my side. Loretta made the quilt that will be at my party. (For the quilt drawing) She was one of the ones who headed up the auction to help us with the medical bills. She didn't blink an eye when she was going all over the place asking even Pepsi and Coke to donate (which they did) I love this gal!

Beside Loretta, sat Ahleesha. The youngest lady in the room. We are "huggin" friends! She calls me Momma Karen. Her hugs and Facebook messages and stuffed peppers helped me through my journey. Ahleesha helped me through one of the hardest days of my life. I didn't want to go to church that day. It was going to be my first day to appear bald at church. I'd have a scarf on but still... unless you've been there, it's hard to know how low you feel at the point where your hair falls out. All of the "it'll grow back" in the world doesn't help at the time.

I had Joe drop me off at the side door because I couldn't face going in the front door and I was too weak to walk from the car. I was going to avoid anyone and everyone and sit in the back. I was late... on purpose. I walked in the side door and around the corner and there was Ahleesha with her big ole hug and tears too. I can't even write this without tears! I'll never forget the love I felt that day and singing on the way home! Thank you girlfriend! I love you and that beautiful family of yours too!!

By Ahleesha, sat Karen S. Karen is like the energizer bunny. She never stops. Karen, ran my sweeper, cleaned my house, made me chicken soup. She brought me bags of ice from Sonic to keep me hydrated. She sat with me until midnight when Joe was on the way home from a job trip. When she found out we were not going to have the tree up last Christmas, she came and put the Christmas tree up and brought wrapped gifts to put under it. Karen was the other half with Loretta who headed up the auction. I have learned a lot from Karen on how to help others. You are dear to me friend! Beside Karen, sat my baby sister Jill.

I love my sister so much and she loves me. She's quiet and steady. EVERY single chemo treatment, she was there for me. She made me a homemade card every treatment and brought it to me along with more pages of the memory book she made for me. She has cleaned my house, decorated for Christmas for me. She even changed her regular day off from work (Monday) to a Tuesday so she could be at chemo with me. Jill & her husband were the first ones that Joe and I told when I was diagnosed. She's never left my side. I can count on my sister, no matter what! I love her to the moon and back. Beside Jill, sat my "kindred spirit" cousin Lois.

Lois herself has had a very difficult year as she had surgery on a tumor on her pituitary gland. It's been a terrible year for her. Lois and I like to laugh and we like to eat.... stuff with sugar in it. We are both fans of coke and chocolate. We also like "pretty things" and parties! But this year we both laid around and sat in our chairs and texted each other. "You ok today? Do you need anything?" (Like either of us could get out to do something for each other!!)

We have cried together and laughed together. We've eaten pizza and desert and popcorn and candy bars all in one setting together. We've looked at the world through a different pair of lenses together this year. No matter how sick she was this year, or how discouraged or afraid she was this year; she would still text me to check on me. We would share dumb brain or boob jokes together and laugh 'til our stitches hurt! I love you Lois! Beside Lois, sat my dear friend Cindy.

Cindy owns the Lords Library in Rolla. She can be serious or laughing in the same minute. I think of her as my encourager!! No matter what it is, she's going to be there for you. I begged her to fill my slot with the bible study group, but she refused saying "No, they were waiting for me (Karen)." That pushed me to keep going, knowing she wasn't giving up on me. I would drop by her store after doctor visits when I'd have the energy and get my hug and she'd give me home made chocolate candy! She probably thought I was dropping by for the candy, but really it was for her encouragement.

Cindy brought me gifts and books at church. I always felt she "had my back" just pushing me to get better because we had more things to do!! Cindy's husband Richard and another friend Joel also kept us in firewood all winter long so Joe didn't have to leave me and cut wood. They are the "bestest"!

Beside Cindy sat Claudia! Claudia has faced both breast cancer and kidney cancer. Claudia is my "hope giver". When Claudia heard I was diagnosed she was there in the seat beside me, praying for me! She spent hours at my house explaining things in a simple way and encouraging me that I could do this and would someday be grateful for the experience. Claudia knew I loved teacups and teapots and at my first chemo she showed up with real china teacups and a pot of tea and sugar cookies. She let me know, I could still have my party right there in the chemo room. She set the pace for the chemo's that would follow. She's still encouraging me and letting me know... "This too shall pass". Everybody needs a friend like Claudia when they ride the bull and I want to be that kind of friend. Beside Claudia and to my left sat Sarah.

Sarah is the lady who threw the luncheon for me. She is a little tiny lady with a heart bigger than herself. She's a "southern lady" with southern style and we can all learn from her. Sarah and her husband Tony have been like rocks to us this year. Sarah gets out of bed when she is sick and waits on people! She is always serving. Even the day of the luncheon she wasn't well and yet, she was still serving people.

This year, she has brought us dinners, and desserts. She has popped in (we live about an hour apart) to drop off a book for me to read or chocolate or cookies or potato soup or pork roast or...... It's not off the shelf for Sarah. Sarah does southern homemade cookin' made with love. I would dare to say, that Sarah might always cook too much, so she'll have some to share.

Sarah has prayed for me and shared her Mississippi friend (Bonnie) with me. She and Tony have text us almost every morning to say... "We prayed for you this morning". What a beautiful lady Sarah is and I'm blessed to have her in my life. I look at these ladies, joining me around a delicious southern meal and the words of that hymn "Look what the Lord has done" sings in my soul!

You may be tired of reading and you may think this is long. However that wasn't the end of my blessing for the day! I'll have to save more for another day as I've got to make my bed!!! I thank God constantly for each of YOU out there. Many more of you could have sat around that table. Both friends and strangers alike who have blessed me over and over this year!!! YOU have blessed me over and over with your encouragement and prayers. I am still struggling with pain from some of the chemo side effects but I'm making progress daily. I'm still pretty good friends with this ole leather recliner and I take my naps. Life isn't like it used to be. In many ways it's better! Come with me my friend.... Let's "grow and glow"!

September 23, 2014

One year ago today; I sat staring at the tears in the eyes of my doctor. I had only met her once before, so her tears surprised me! She was talking Greek or Gibberish or something like that. I'm not sure, because actually I wasn't even hearing what she had to say. Only two things registered with me.... the tears in her eyes and the words she had just said to me. "You have cancer!"

I wasn't surprised at her words. After all I was there and "peeked" when the computer was spitting out all kinds of images. I knew enough about the symptoms that caused me to scurry to the doctor when I knew I had them. (The symptoms) I also knew that when you are rushed straight to a mammogram, then a biopsy with titanium bits for markers put in you "just in case you have surgery" and a "just in case" introduction to the cancer navigator nurse, all in one afternoon.... that there was a more than likely chance there was a problem. No.... I wasn't surprised but I was SHOCKED. I know I was shocked because I didn't say anything to her. I just stared at her and wondered about the tears in her eyes. (How bad is this, that my doctor has tears in her eyes?) Unless you have been there, you can't imagine how it feels to hear those harsh words (no matter how tenderly they are spoken). Your brain stops (& I'm not sure when if ever it picks up again).

Coming Full Circle Makes Me Dizzy!

As you all know... it has been a year like no other for me! I have endured sixteen chemo treatments, two surgeries, thirty-six radiation treatments, and I can't even count how many shots and blood draws. I have endured needles where needles should never be! I have endured losing my hair, my eyelashes and eyebrows. I have lost body parts and my figure.

I also lost twenty pounds though with chocolate and ice cream; I have managed to gain ten of it back. I have endured both chemo taste and chemo brain. I have slept days in a row and been awake just as many. I have endured dust on my furniture and cobwebs in my thinking. There are days when I can't figure out my left hand from my right hand (literally) I have wept until I had no tears left. I have had days when I literally wanted to just stay in bed and cover my head until... oh maybe next week!

I have ridden the bull, fought the monster and slayed the dragon. I have WON!!!!! I am now considered to be a ONE year survivor!!! Though this has truly been the hardest year of my life, I have been blessed more than I knew blessing could flow.

God has blessed me with more friends than I can count. You who have cheered me on, encouraged me and prayed for me. You have sent me cards, letters, messages, text and gifts of all kind. You have dropped by my house with meals and cookies, and books and candies. You have come by to just encourage me or check on me or offer to help. You've brought firewood and offerings, blankets and hugs.

I have been cheered on by three year olds to 90 year olds! You have cried with me and laughed with me! You have not given up on me! Even now as I am recovering, you are still here for me! I thank each of you for what you have taught me! For the hugs, the cheers, the help.

I look back over this year and know it was a rough one, one I never want to repeat. But more than the rough spots, I see your smiling faces. I feel your prayers. I feel your pushes and your tugs, your "you can do this"! That's what I remember the most.

God never left my side and YOU were there for me!! I hate being slow, but every day, I feel like I'm getting better! I'm ready for better already!!! My survivor "thank you party" is almost here! We're going to have a balloon lift off. Our color theme is going to be "orange-yellow-red-green-blue"! I love color and when those balloons lift to the skies, they are going to represent LIFE! Bright and beautiful! I hope YOU can be there as YOU are a part of what makes my life beautiful.

September 29th, 2014

I'm glad we've got a little sunshine back in the house! Thing Two has come to spend the night with us. I can hardly believe it's the same little girl who spent so much time with us the last three years before I was diagnosed. We have missed both Thing One and Thing Two so much! She was one excited little girl tonight and chattered the whole way here.

We were backing out of her parents drive when I looked over at Poppa Joe and said.... "I do believe we have a little girl in our back seat!" She popped up and said... "It's ME!!!! Melody! I'm going home with you!!!" She proceeded to chatter with updates on her life. What letter she was learning in school. The fact that she loves "Jimmy" and they play house at preschool. She takes a nap and has a pillow and a cot... etc. etc. etc.

Joe asked her if she could say her ABC's and she started singing right away. A B C D E F G....H I J K lellooooow m o p........ etc. Now I know my ABC's next time won't you sing with me! Joe pops up and says.... "Sure! We'll sing with you!" So we start in.... she chimes in too! When we finish she says... "MAN! You guys are GREAT at this! Let's do it again!" And that's how we managed to sing our ABC's several times on the way home.

She was so excited when she saw the words again on our door: "Nana's Happy House!" We played "cooking" once we got here and Poppa Joe and I were the customers. We drank "girl milk and boy milk". (This all depends on the color of the container it's poured out of!!!) Playing "cooking" is real similar to "restaurant" except we never got a bill and we left our tip in Yankee dimes!

It was time to get ready for bed and I looked around at how quickly things had got out of place. I wondered aloud... "I wonder who messed this room up!" She said... "YOU and I did Nana! You'll have to help me clean it up!" Just like she marveled that I didn't already know that!

She started out in her own little bed, but decided that she needed me to lay down with her so she could go to sleep. Since I'm too big for the little toddler bed we laid down on Thing Two's big bed. I closed my eyes! Her hands went all over my face! All over my short hair! At one time... she had her feet with her toes on my head! "Ouch Mels! That hurts!" "Oh that hurts you??? I was just tickling your head with my toes!"

I keep my eyes shut and she cuddles down again. I must have got a ton of kisses on my face... my arms... my hands... my head. A hundred "I love you"! At one point she took a hold of my hand and placed her little hand in mine and said in my ear... "You are my best friend". My heart smiled, but I kept my eyes shut! It took an hour and I fell asleep before she did.... but she's out now! Ah yes.... there's sunshine in the house tonight! It feels like things are getting back to normal!!!

Poppa Joe has a "problem"! Though he came up with the idea to grow his beard, racing me in growing my hair, he really hasn't taken to the beard idea as much I have! He's been itching for some time to shave. Since Thing One and Thing Two have been excited about this competition, I suggested he shouldn't shave without consulting with them first. At first they were both all for his shaving but the more they thought about it, they switched sides!!!

Thing One informed him in no uncertain terms... "This is a competition and if you shave now you will lose!!!" He really doesn't want to lose since Thing One has also stated what the prize for the winner will be!!! Lots of cuddles from Thing One and Thing Two!!! Ahhh yes.... Poppa Joe has a "problem"!!!! Tee hee!!!

CHAPTER 14

Time to Kick My Heels Up & Pay It Forward

October 3rd, 2014

How about that!!!! I got my first haircut today! That's another step towards normal!!! Thanks Tatum for trimming me up a bit!!!

October 18th, 2014

Things are looking up! My Doctor changed me from the first five year chemo pill to a new one. Thirty days on that pill was just about to change my personality! I have only had two of the new one so far, but I'm already feeling so much better not taking the first one. I was feeling like I was back on a lower dose of chemo. I was not a happy camper. I had aches and pains and desperate feelings. My heart cried… "Oh my FIVE years of feeling like THIS!!!" I'm so hoping this little white pill does better. Who knew things could be so complicated!! I thought "done was done"!!! On the upside, I'm so looking forward to my survivor thank you party in just a week! I am so ready to "PAR-TAAAAY"

October 22, 2014

It feels so good to accomplish something I've wanted to complete this year! I have finished up the prayer wall!!! I hope I haven't left someone's name off. I have been so blessed to be praying for you all this year and to have you praying for me! THANK YOU!!!!!

October 24th, 2014

Oh how excited I am! We've been looking forward to this party ever since we announced it! I hope I can sleep tonight as I am overwhelmed at the response to this celebration!!! We have a super day planned and are excited for each of you who can make it!! The prayer wall is done, quilt is hung for the drawing (I hope you win) Cakewalk cakes coming.... Wally's BBQ pulled pork smells GREAT! Mints, cupcakes and cookies etc. ready. The balloons are ready to be blown up in the morning. The games are ready and the music lined up. Eggs for the egg toss ready. I think even the mules and the little donkey is excited! OH I can't wait! Thank you Jill for being at my side every step of the way on preparing for this party! I'm feeling excited!!

October 25th, 2014

What a wonderful survival celebration thank you party! We had almost a hundred balloons of all colors blown up. The decorations were beautiful out at the Mule Barn. Wally's BBQ made you hungry as you walked in the room. Cakes and cookies and a long row of tables filled with food ran down the center of the room. Our musicians played and sang all afternoon. What beautiful music! I loved every minute of it.

This was our party to thank each of you and our community for standing by us and supporting us so much this past year. We truly would not have made it this past experience without each of you. Every one of you are near and dear to our hearts! Thank you for each of you who attended!!

We had cake walks with yummy cakes to be won. Each cake was made and donated by friends of ours! We had expected to just have about a four hour party. However there was so much fun riding the mules and the little donkey that we ended up serving again for supper and didn't leave there until after 10 p.m. What a wonderful day!

Tonight... I'm tired to the bone and blessed more than I ever realized. I love you each!!! Besides the music, the food, the cake walk, the mule rides and donkey ride and games, I do believe my favorite part was watching the two balloon lift offs. Beautiful, colorful balloons filling the skies representing LIFE! I Love the prayer wall also. Jill and I worked hard on this wall and it now hangs in my house as a reminder of each of you who have been praying me through this journey! Thank you so much for your prayers and continued support!

October 29th, 2014

One year ago today; I was up bright and early so wishing it was any day except "October 29th 2013! It was my first ride on that ole mean bull and I was scared spitless. It's been a long journey, a hard journey, but one with blessings and an over flowing cup!

I lost my hair, my eyelashes, my eyebrows, my breast, my fingernails and toenails, my strength, and my babysitting time with Thing One and Thing Two. There were times, I felt like I'd almost lost my mind! Most of the time, I spent right here in my ole recliner, too exhausted to move.

I couldn't grocery shop, or walk any distance. Others cooked for Joe and me and cleaned our house. To date, it has been the hardest year of my life. That being said... I did not lose my sense of humor, nor did I lose my confidence in God. I gained so much more this past year than I lost!

When I first started my journey, a friend told me, that I would come out on the other end a different person. That I have done for sure! It would be impossible to write all of the things and people that I am so thankful for!

I have learned to reach across the aisle! I have shared my story with complete strangers and listened to theirs. I have cried with you and you have cried with me! I am most grateful that I did not have to take this journey alone! You have walked with me every step of the way. When I have been self-absorbed with my pain or too tired to take another step, you have sat with me and listened and rested.

I have learned that even though pain makes one feel it's all about them; it really isn't. I have learned that I can grow through your pain and you can grow through mine! I have learned that people have hearts of gold and are sweeter than honey! I have learned, there is always someone sicker than I am and who has less than me. I have learned the cup is not half full but is always overflowing! I have learned to rest and sip from the overflow!

I have learned who makes the overflow! I would never want to repeat this year, nor would I wish this year on anyone else, but I'm grateful that my biggest fear did not materialize. I was so afraid, I would not learn what I was supposed to learn though this journey. I did learn! In fact, I would say, I learned more than I ever wanted to learn.

I have learned that people care! I am constantly being asked questions. Like..."Your hair looks cute like that; are you going to keep it short?" NO! NO! NO! (With a smile) I want hair! One day it will be long again! One day it will blow in the wind again!!!

Here's another one... "Are you going to have reconstructive surgery?" Nope! There are several reasons why I've made this decision. Number one being, my doctor told me with as deep as my surgery was, that reconstruction surgery would probably have me dealing with more and more surgeries and issues because of the problems that would arise from reconstructive surgery. (In my case)

Number two... I'm tired of surgeries, needles and being poked at. I'm also afraid of it! It's going to take a lot of courage for me to go under the knife again when I get my port out (whenever that is)

The Pink Duck

I'm going to "pioneer for the flat chested" ladies. You can always say..."You knew me when.....!" I'm ok with my decision and so is my Joe! Which brings me to something else I'm grateful for!

I'm grateful for "My Joe". I've always called him "My Joe" and he's always called me his "girl"! My Joe has carried me this year and he has not grown weary of it and I have certainly been a heavy load. He has planted kiss after kiss on my bald head. He has held me when I've cried buckets of tears and he has wiped my cheeks. He has promised me that I'm the most beautiful gal in the world to him (even bald). He's proven it over and over with his kindness and caring ways. I thank God for him every day!

I also thank God for each of you! As I look at my prayer wall, I can't stop the tears of gratefulness that slip down my cheeks. I just don't know anyone who is more blessed than me!

That 'ole bull and I had some words! We did some violent rounds and he 'near "skeert me ta death", but I WON! He's been put out 'ta pasture! I conquered the radiation monster and slayed the dragon (standing on one foot with one hand behind my back)!

Actually I was flat on my back, praying your names over and over so I wouldn't panic when that three foot thick door sealed me in the room alone! I've celebrated and lifted a hundred balloons in the sky!

I still fall on my face and thank God for each of you who have prayed me through this year, whether it's been one time or you're still praying! I know God heard your prayers and I know because of you, He answered and I am here today, anxious to kick up my heels! Most of all, I thank God for his mercies! For his still small voice that said to me... "I know the plans I have for you, plans to prosper you and not to harm you, plans to give you hope and a future." (Jeremiah 9:11)

I am thankful that all through the storm we can hold onto HIM! That he never lets us go! I hope that whatever season you are going through that you will know Christ as your savior, that you will seek His face in all you do and trust HIM! Thank you my friend for traveling this journey with me! I love you!!

Chapter 15

Thanksgiving

November 1st, 2014

How I love this month!!! The month of Thanksgiving and a time to reflect on all we are thankful for! Day One and I am thankful for my wonderful husband! He has always loved me and I him! But this year has been sweeter than ever before! He has carried me as I've been too weak to help myself. No matter what I've needed or asked for, he has jumped hoops to make sure I am taken care of and at ease.

    I thank God every day for this man! A man, I dated just almost two months before marrying! How blessed I am!!! I thank God that my man is a godly man. I am thankful he is a praying man and a bible reading man! I am thankful that God is first with him and I am second! I am proud to stand by my man, to walk hand in hand! This month we will be married 39 years! Yes! I'm thankful for my Joe!

November 2nd, 2014

Day 2 of Thanksgiving! I had two sisters!!! One I referred to as my big sister (even though she really was a little thing) and one who I always refer to as my baby sister! There's nothing quite like a sister. We were like three peas in a pod. Even though we don't look alike or even act alike for that matter. One look at us and you can tell we're sisters.

Now, Lynn was the crafty one. She made beautiful handmade crafts and my home still treasures many of them! Lynn and I used to call each other up and race cleaning our homes. We'd go for the kitchen and then call each other up to make sure we'd both got our jobs done. Then we'd work on the living room... call each other....etc. Since we lived in different states, we also wrote letters.

Before Lynn died, she gave me a package of all of the letters I'd written her through the years. She had saved everyone for me because she knew one day I'd like to reread them because they were chalk full of stories of my three boys growing up! I'll miss my sister until I see her again. She certainly was the best big sister ever!

Now Jill was my baby sister!! We also had a routine of cleaning together. Only we would get us a notebook and fill it up with everything in the house that needed to be done and then start at the top and start cleaning and crossing things off the list! We both can probably run across a notebook with a list of chores needed to be done with half the list crossed off at any given time!

Jill has a way with words! She says her words backwards and rhymes everything. Jill is the queen of little things! Little sayings, little gifts and little things she delights in doing for you and you delight in receiving! When I was going through chemo, she would make me a handmade card with a poem or cute saying in it every chemo session. She even made me one on the times I wasn't able to take chemo. She'd bring me little gifts.... like a pink ink pen, or pink socks or a scarf, candy or a balloon. There's no better little sister then my baby sister!

We three girls grew up dressing alike, and singing our hearts out together. I don't think we ever did dishes without singing and I know we never went on a trip without singing all the way there and back. I'm so thankful for my two sisters and that I was placed right smack dab in between the two of them. I got the best of both sides!!! Thank you God for both of my sisters!!

November 3rd, 2014

Day 3 of Thanksgiving! Hum 3... What to write… What to write... Ah! How about, "My three sons!" Yep, that's it! I don't know of a mother anywhere who loves her children more than I love my three sons! Three ornery, full of fun and life sons! Yep! That's what our home was full of! It's amazing how full three sons can fill up a house or the backseat of a car for that matter!

Every time a nurse placed a perfect little boy in my arms, I was amazed and full of love! Never in my life was I prepared for or expected to have 3 sons! It certainly was "on the job" training for me! Our sons were fun, funny and smart. They each brought our home joy beyond our wildest imaginations!

Our oldest son is Timothy! Ah the stories I could tell on Timothy Weber. Arriving in this world at a whopping 4 pounds and 8 ounces, Timothy wasn't even as big as his daddy's arm! We called him "short shanks" forever! He's now a big guy about 6'3"!! Maybe more! Timothy lives in North Dakota where he works with the oil fields and we haven't seen him for a couple of years. I miss him more and more everyday along with his four beautiful children.

Timothy and I used to spend hours lying on the floor on our tummies playing Skip-Bo and other games! Next time he comes home... I'm going to beat him at a hand of Kanasta!!! He has a beautiful voice and I love to hear him especially sing..."I've been everywhere man!" Sometimes when he calls me, we'll end up singing parts of songs together. I miss harmonizing with him. Timothy has the best bear hugs ever and I can't wait for another one from him!

Son #2 is our son Wes Weber. Wes was our "full of life and loving it" son! Bright eyed and attracted to anything that had flashing lights or moved! Oh the stories we could share about Wes! He was a happy, happy child and his school principal asked me once if Wesley was always happy! He was....

except when he wasn't! Wes is steady, dependable and always checking on his mom and dad! (That would be Joe and me)

We raised our sons while owning a lumber yard and sawmill. Two of our three sons loved the lumber business! Wesley was not one of those two. From a little tyke, he was determined to be in law enforcement and law. Every goal he has set in those fields so far, he has accomplished or is on his way to accomplishing! I love his visits home, he and I always get a night of staying up and talking until the wee hours of the morning! That is my favorite time with Wes. I can't wait to see him again and get my big old bear hug! Wes will reach another of his goals when he graduates from Washburn Law School this coming May of 2015.

When Wes was about 3, the doctor told me that I would probably never have any more children! A month later, I was expecting Son #3. Now there's some good stories about James too, but I'm well aware that all three of my sons could spill the beans on me too so I'm keeping quite! I know.... aww shucks! We always referred to James or "Jake" as we call him, as our sunshine! He came along at a difficult time in our life (the in sickness or health time with Joe) and he was such a happy little ball of sunshine. He was also a clown by nature. We home schooled him after the sixth grade but from K through 5th, I don't think he had a teacher that didn't let me know he was the class clown. I was never sure if I was supposed to do anything about that or not! (As if I could!) He still can be a clown. A long tall, 6'4" clown! He can keep us laughing! (A gift all three of our boys possessed really)

Jake and I share our birthday month. We always went birthday shopping together and while he was growing up, went on several trips together. I always felt he "had my back!" He's told me several times that I'm one of his best friends and I keep that tucked down in my heart! James like Wes is in law school so I expect one of these days he'll be smarter than me! Huh Jake?? He will graduate December of 2015.

We absolutely LOVED raising our three sons. There were many, many challenges and lots and lots of laughter and fun.

Thanksgiving

Dinner time at our table was always the best ever with lots of "can you top this?" and "cut it out boys!" There was never a dull moment! There's a lot I would like a "do over" on, of course but one thing I wouldn't trade for anything in the world and that's having these three young men call me "Mom"! In fact.... I think it's about time they do call me!!! I love them each with all of my heart and I thank God every day that HE chose ME to be their mama!!! Yep... "Life is bright... we have three sons!"

November 4th, 2014

Well I'm a day behind on my thankful post, but I did not want to "short change" the FOUR I wanted to mention for day four! I wanted to tell you about four people who have really impacted not only my life, but the life of Joe and our sons. Those four people would be Joe's parents (Joe & Mary) and my parents (Roy & Alice) I'll start with Joe's dad (Joe SR).

Joe SR has been gone from this world 28 years! He was a pretty quiet man with heart problems. He'd had open heart surgery the year before Joe and I met and married. I never felt like I really knew him all that well but I do have some wonderful memories of him. Joe SR was a truck gardener. Instead of planting a row of strawberries, he'd plant an acre! I have never seen such huge, juicy strawberries.

Joe SR taught my husband work ethics. He was a hard worker. He was also a good husband to his wife. I remember Joe's uncle telling me when I became engaged to Joe that if he treated me half as good as his dad had treated his mother, I wouldn't have any complaints! Joe SR took me to the grocery store one time and told me I could have anything I wanted. I do believe he was a little shocked when the only thing I wanted was popcorn. I'll never forget his laugh! Who knows, after telling me that...he may have been relieved!

He also had a little tune he always sang. He couldn't carry much of a tune. He would just sing out once in a while.... "DO,DO,DO,DO,dooo,doooo"! Every once in a while I still burst out with the same funny little tune in memory of him. He was a

The Pink Duck

good man and I am grateful for the way he raised my husband teaching him how to be a good dad and a wonderful husband.

Number 2 on my list tonight is my mother-in-law, Mary. I was married several years before I realized my mother-in-law wasn't bigger than me! She was 4'10 or 11" and feisty! (I'm 5'6") She was thrilled when I married Joe because at the ripe ole age of 23, she didn't think Joe was ever going to marry! Well, he did and we did it up right tight!

Mary was the kind of grandmother who liked to tell her grandkids stories. They would try to sit on her lap and complain that she didn't really have a lap because she was so short. Mary was a godly woman and I loved to hear her give her testimony at church. She had a great understanding of the bible and could always feed you from it.

She was also a good cook. In fact she taught me how to make the best fried chicken north of the border. She also taught me how to make homemade noodles. She made the best donuts and fruitcakes!!! Mary and I traveled a lot together and had a lot of fun. She's been gone almost four years now and I miss her. She's the only person I know who has ever backed over herself with a car and lived to tell it!!

I'm thankful for my mother-in-law. She could be a pickle sometimes and at times I wanted to bop her! But I always loved her and respected her as my husband's mother and am forever in her debt for my wonderful husband.

My own parents were completely different than Joe's family. Let me count the ways! Joe's parents had goats and geese and cats and dogs and pigs. We had gold fish once, maybe twice. My folks are city folks, Joe's folks were country all the way! With all of the differences, our parents still loved each other and had great respect for the others.

Number 3 on my list today is my dad. My dad was strict. I have to say that first in case he reads this. He would fall into the tall, dark and handsome category. I can't count how many of my girlfriends got a crush on my dad. Dad is completely organized and has a system for everything. We grew up with him remodeling homes. He'd buy one, remodel it, sell it and we'd have to move again. He loved to garden and no matter where we lived, he'd want to go on a walk after dinner and "tour da farm"! (Remember we lived in the city!!) Our yard was always "the back forty"!

He was a good provider. He took us on vacations and always saw to it that we'd saved up for "fun stuff" before we left so we didn't ask him for money on the trip. We three girls drove our dad nuts singing "I'm a little piece of tin" on road trips. We would start the song with the letter B... singing "B'm b bittle biece of bin, bobody boes bhat abides bith in......" and head down the alphabet. I don't think we ever got past the letter "D" before he'd shut us up and we'd pass sneaky grins at one another. We always tried to see how far we could get with the song before he'd clamp us down! He did love to hear us sing though just not that song!

I appreciate my dad more and more every day! He just celebrated his 84th birthday and we're blessed to have him!

Last but not least is my mother! Her name is Alice but family calls her "Wydie"! Now my mother was a character! As beautiful as my dad was handsome! She was red headed with a personality to match. She was the movement in the room! She was super strict too, but she also loved to play! She loved summer because we kids were home from school. She played games with us and was constantly playing tricks on us! I can't tell you how many times I've got wet from one of her tricks.

Mom never worked outside of the home. She kept a neat and tidy ship. She played the piano and the guitar and I probably can't remember a day without music in our home growing up. We had either popcorn or ice cream almost every night as a bedtime snack! Mom spent a lot of time on her knees praying. She still reads her bible a LOT. I am grateful for the influence she has been on my life. I thank God for these four godly people and for their commitment on teaching each of their children about God. I hope I can be half the parent these four were. I love each of them!

The Pink Duck

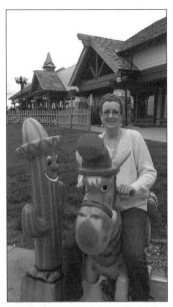

I'm making progress! I think I can handle this little guy! Anybody have a quarter?

November 13th, 2014

Day 13 of Thanksgiving!!! I am thankful for GREAT Doctor reports!!! I went today for my port flush and blood test...again!! Of course these reports are all GREEK to me! I was sitting there looking over the numbers and my doctor was so excited she kept repeating "These are good!!! Look at these numbers!!!" The room was small so I couldn't turn a cartwheel! Of course, I couldn't turn one down the hall either... too many people there!! I couldn't even turn one outside because it was too cold! However I AM happy about my results! She also let me loose to go back on my Melaleuca cell wise which helps build good cells back! Happy! Happy! Happy! Hillary Bleckman and Stephanie Brown Pritchett I needed you during the port flush! Yep... you guessed it... I've given so much blood this past year that Nicole couldn't get any blood from it. Good thing she's cheerful and I like her!!! Missed you Julie Lange Terry Here's calling you back to the Bond Clinic!!!

Chapter 16

Chicken Soup & Pink Ducks

December 7th 2014

How does one share a "chicken soup for the soul" type of moment? I have rolled this around in my mind all week, wondering how to share. Wondering if I should, knowing that I must. After all you have been on this journey over a year with me. I know you are still praying for me as I am for you. I have been healing and even though I'm certainly not back to what I call normal, I am making progress.

That being said, I suffer with neuropathy in both my feet and hands from the chemo. It's frustrating to say the least. If you aren't familiar with that, let me share. It's like you can feel your bones in your feet when you walk and you are numb and in pain with thousands of needles poking you. As my dad said, you feel like you are walking on bubble wrap. Problem is... there's no bubbles to pop so it's not much fun. You feel every thread in your socks and it's painful. I have trouble writing with my hands because of the nerve damage. It's hard to hang onto an ink pen or even type for that matter. I had to get my wedding band resized because of swelling.

My mind is finally feeling like it is clearing more though I still am having trouble with my spelling (& sleeping). Other things are clearer than I remembered before. It's a crazy new normal. The other day I decided... "Enough is enough" and

I'm going to go to the chiropractor in spite of wearing this "port" (which I hate).

It was a big deal to me because I knew medically this wasn't something my doctor wanted me to do just yet because of the port. (Which I hate) There is the concern of it being damaged or in my mind flying loose and coming undone However, sitting in a recliner for most of a year, I was desperate to get to my chiropractor and see if I could get some pain relief (without medication). Anxious to go but scared spitless because of this ole port (which I hate).

My chiropractor assured me he had adjusted many patients with ports and I did not doubt his ability. I roped (I learned that while bull riding) Joe into going with me, just in case there was a problem and the port (which I hate) did accidently come loose and cause blood to fly all over the room and make a mess and I might have to go to the hospital and have them cut on me again and they'd have to sew me up again and give me more shots (which I hate too). They would have to mop the floor at the chiropractors etc. etc. etc. My imagination was locked into full speed ahead, but I was determined to get the adjustment in spite of my fears about my port (which I hate) accidently coming loose.

So there we sat and the doctor came in to adjust my aching back. I was just about as tense as one could be. Now for those of you who have never gone to a chiropractor and received an adjustment, let me assure you, it isn't in anyway a bad experience normally. You stand on a moving table machine thingy and the doctor pushes a button and you end up lying face down on the table with your face planted in a padded crack on the table. (How am I doing so far?? Can you see it??)

Just about the time I got settled down there where my port (which I hate) wasn't pinching into my chest, the doctor began using some modern machine on me that targets the different areas and a lines your spine and straightens your back. My face is down in the face crack (I'm sure DR Powell) has the proper words for all of these, but I'm from the old school where it's "poppin and crackin". (Sorry Doctor) I can't "see" anything but I can feel and hear.

I hear a scuffling of several feet and feel three then four hands on me. I pause in my panic mode and count the hands.... I recounted... One...two...three.... Now my doctor has a new partner which I've never met and I thought..."That's funny, Doctor must be a little nervous or cautious too since he's brought his partner in with him!" I thought it odd that he didn't introduce me to him before working with me. It was like his hand was on me to steady me and comfort me. (Maybe even to keep me on the table, or as I thought... help in case my port (which I hate) did come flying loose.

Doctor finished with the machine and I "flopped" over with my eyes still closed and he adjusted me again. I felt a bit weepy just from the stress of being afraid of being adjusted with the port (which I hate) in and the doctor left the room to let me rest a minute. Joe came over and held my hand too sooth me and let me know he was supporting me once again!

I hope you are still with me, because the good part is yet to come. We left and headed for the house, my port (which I hate) still intact and my posture feeling better. I mentioned to Joe about DR Powell's new partner coming in and wondered why DR Powell didn't introduce him to us. Joe said...."There wasn't another doctor in the room, Karen!"

I thought a minute and said... "Oh, so it was you who had your hand on me....thanks for that, it really helped!" Joe said... "What do you mean?" I explained about feeling his hand on me while the doctor was running the machine on me. I said... "I counted the hands on me and there was three one time and then four!" Joe said.... "Karen, I never touched you until the doctor left, I sat there in the corner and watched him adjust you!"

I don't know about you... but I even have goose bumps telling you about it. We were both quite for a bit, looking at each other with a stunned deer in the headlight look on our faces, then Joe said... "Haven't we been praying that God would have HIS hand on you? That was God you felt!"

Oh MY.... how does one comprehend that?? How does one even share??? I have heard many of you pray this past year that God would have his hand on me! THANK YOU! I have also prayed this for you!!! May the peace that passes all understanding be yours! May you know God's hand upon your life! May you snuggle in the shelter of His wings! May you not just believe IN God but may you BELIEVE God!

I thank God that He answers our prayers!! He will never leave us nor forsake us!! Scripture tells us that we are the apple of God's eye! Don't ya just want to be the twinkle in HIS eye!!! I know I do!

December 21st, 2014

I have wondered several times how and when I should end this book. The problem is, my story has not ended (of which I'm very grateful for)! I'm still adapting to this five year pill. I have days which I find it very hard to walk. Some days, I can however even skip! Today I climbed up on chairs and helped my mother redecorate her kitchen. Not for anything would I dare let her know how hard it is for me to climb up and off of a chair. Knowing her, she would insist on climbing on the chairs and doing it herself! She is after all 39 years young plus tax and shipping. That adds up to 81 years old! It was my pleasure to help her!

I still get my words backwards sometimes and can't figure out my left from right other times. Humor helps in times like that! My bones ache and the neuropathy bothers me terrible at times. I'm not happy with my shape or how slow I am. I'm really excited that I'm getting my hair back. It's not the same color and it's not straight like it was. But its hair and that makes me happy.

Thing One does not like gray hair! We've had this conversation before. I had not seen her in a while and she was excited that my hair was growing! She scrunched up her face and asked "Nana are you going to have gray hair?" Knowing how she feels about gray hair; I said..."It's going to be black and white!!!!" Her face lit up and she said..."OOOOooooooOOOOO!!!!

So often people ask, "What can I do to help?" There is so much you can do. Sometimes people stay away because they don't know what to say or do. I'm sure you got some ideas while reading this book. I was not used to being helped as I like to be the helper! I learned a lot from those who jumped in and helped.

When you are going through Chemo, you are very sick and very aware that things aren't getting done. When someone says they want to help, it is a big relief. Run the sweeper, dust, fix meals and drop them off. Jumping in and doing the dishes is a big help. Helping with the laundry (but only things like towels unless you're asked to do more). Remember it is still the other person's home and private domain. Don't clean out the fridge without asking.

If you are bringing a meal, find out what the patient can eat. Potato soup was one thing I could eat. My poor husband was grateful when something was delivered besides potato soup. Yes, do consider the caregiver too. They have a full plate being a caregiver. Disposable dishes are the best so the patient doesn't have to try to remember where the dishes go back to. They are exhausted keeping up too! Ice cream and a bag of ice from Sonic was a couple of my favorite items!

A card is always appropriate with a note or letter. It's ok to say, "I don't know what to say, but I'm thinking of you!" A phone call is very much appreciated before showing up. Other times, if you are close to the patient, dropping in with a surprise batch of cookies just might be the thing that makes the patients day! A box of candy or flowers are always appreciated. A cozy blanket is much appreciated because you are cold a lot when you take chemo. I even received a nice pair of pajamas which I appreciated because I spent a lot of time in my jammies.

I would caution against giving a lot of "pink" cancer gifts. I do realize this is the breast cancer theme. However, most patients aren't going to be decorating in this theme and during recovery receiving more pink clothing and items can make one feel like others still feel like they have the disease. Most are seriously wanting to move beyond this point and getting on to normal again.

If someone has decided to take chemo, don't tell them horror stories of why they shouldn't and don't give them books on what they need to do different. They are under professional care with someone who has studied their blood work and worked with their labs. Everyone is different and what might work for one, may not work with another. I was given the choice of chemo or going natural. My chances of survival weren't as great going natural as taking chemo. I was at a stage where I didn't have time to wait on going natural to work. It wasn't my choice but it was the wisest choice for me. It might not be for you or your relative. Whatever a person chooses, encourage them to follow their doctors' advice. Many don't know that you can't always mix natural with medications. There should be no guilt in whatever plan of survival one chooses.

Sitting with one or driving them to and from the doctors can be a huge help. We appreciated gifts of gas cards. Short visits and short phone calls are welcome. We received several cards from one sweet little lady who attends our church. How encouraging those cards were to me! I even received cards from strangers telling me they were praying for me. Friendships were formed. I even had a couple of friends who dared to send me funny cards! They delighted me! The gift I received the most of and appreciated the most was the continued prayers. Knowing others were praying helped me though many a bull ride and trips to the doctors. Always pray!

I went to a support group yesterday! Actually, the invitation sounded more like a party, so I went! My eyes are now opened! I sat in a room with possibly 25 - 30 ladies. We went around the room to introduce ourselves. It sounded somewhat like this.... "My name is___, I'm from___, I was diagnosed with stage __ cancer on (date)". WOW what a beautiful group of ladies, diagnosed anywhere from 11 - 14 years ago to just diagnosed this week!" What a group of courageous, victorious women! I truly was amazed as I watched each woman introduce herself. It left me breathless and I could hardly wait to hear each story! I wanted the details! When you are diagnosed with cancer, all of a sudden... you feel a bit like the adulterous woman who had to wear the big red letter "A" on her chest. Instead ours is a big pink C plastered on our chest, our forehead, our heart and every tee-shirt stuffed in the back of our closet! You feel like it sticks out like a sore thumb and for sure you can't drop it from your mind! The feeling gets worse as you lose your hair, your eye lashes and fingernails. You even see yourself as different. You look for the real you! The one who doesn't cry at the drop of a hat. Who has energy to boot and never wallows in self-pity!

Listening to each lady made me feel normal again! In this room of beautiful women, I was just like everyone else. A conqueror, a battle scarred conqueror! These women had climbed mountains and stood and sang their song at the top! Oh how they gave me courage!! I was no longer different from everyone else. In this room, I was one and the same!

Do you know that we're ALL bald? Yep, I'm talking about you and me! Just try removing your hair and see what's underneath! Yep... just bald! Do you know... right under that bald is where your attitude is stored? Just a thought.... I'm glad Carol Walter invited me to this group. If you have a battle of any kind that you are fighting, I'd encourage you to find a group to join. They will help you and you will help them. It's more about where we're going, then where we've been. A big step in moving forward! Sometimes we get "stuck in our pain". A group can help you move beyond that. Did you know pain can become an addiction? The birds are singing, the sun is shining....time to step out!

I want to end my book by encouraging each of you to get your exams EARLY! Don't keep putting it off like I did. In the long run; it isn't worth it! PLEASE go get your exam! Order you a pink duck and put it in your shower where you will be reminded to do your breast exam monthly! Encourage your spouse to do his exam too! Buy a package of pink ducks and pass them out to your family and friends! Help me put one in every home in America! Let's beat this beast and put those ole bulls out to pasture for keeps!

Away with the dragons and monsters! Be proactive with your health!

Second, I would like to encourage each of you to learn about Jesus and what he has done for you! Accept Him as your personal Savior. Ask Him into your heart and life. Let Him change your life! Facing anything in life no matter how difficult is so much easier with Him at your side. Celebrating with Him at your side is so much easier also! Remember that I love you each and I thank you for reading my story! I hope it has inspired you in some way. I hope maybe you got a few belly laughs. If it has encouraged you in anyway, I hope you will share it. Thank you and May God bless you abundantly!

To follow my story, you can find me on face book at Karen's Cancer Kickin Crew

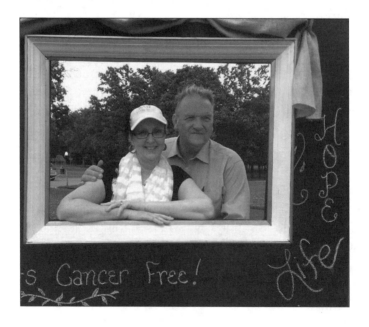